PHARMACEUTICAL SAFETY WITHDRAWALS

PHARMACEUTICAL SAFETY WITHDRAWALS

A Comparative Study of the United States and Canada

Dominika A. Jegen

\<teneo\> // press

YOUNGSTOWN, NEW YORK

This book is dedicated to my grandparents, Janina and Stefan Przyszlak, whose passion for their family, support for education, and love for others inspire me daily. You are incredible and greatly loved.

Apart from those who make science, who study it, who defend it or who submit to it, there exist, fortunately, a few people either trained as scientists or not, who open the black boxes [facts] so that outsiders may have a glimpse at them.
—Bruno Latour (1987, p. 15)

TABLE OF CONTENTS

LIST OF FIGURES

LIST OF ABBREVIATIONS

ADHD	attention deficit hyperactivity disorder
AIDS	acquired immunodeficiency syndrome
ANT	actor network theory
COMT	catechol-o-methyltransferase enzyme
COX-2	cyclooxygenase-II enzyme
DIN	drug identification number
DNA	deoxyribonucleic acid
DSI	Division of Scientific Investigations (U.S.)
FDA	Food and Drug Administration
HPFB	Health Products and Food Branch (Canada)
ICH	International Conference on Harmonization of Technical Requirements for Registration of Pharmaceuticals for Human Use
IFPMA	International Federation of Pharmaceutical Manufacturers and Associations

IND	investigational new drug
IOM	Institute of Medicine (U.S.)
NDA	new drug application
NOC	notice of compliance
PDUFA	Prescription Drug User Fee Act (U.S.)
PhRMA	Pharmaceutical Research and Manufacturers of America
U.S.	United States
WHO	World Health Organization

PHARMACEUTICAL SAFETY WITHDRAWALS

INTRODUCTION

In 2004 the public was shocked to learn that Vioxx® (rofecoxib), a popular anti-inflammatory drug, had been in widespread use for 5 years, even though the drug nearly doubled the risk of myocardial infarction and stroke in patients, and was documented to have this effect in preapproval clinical trials. Its withdrawal from the market in the United States provoked serious doubts about the adequacy of the Food and Drug Administration's (FDA) drug-safety surveillance system (Avorn, 2007). During the same year, the FDA approved the drug Ketek® (telithromycin), praising it as the first of a new class of antimicrobial agents to circumvent antibiotic resistance. "Since then, Ketek has been linked to dozens of cases of severe liver injury, been the subject of a series of progressively more urgent safety warnings, and sparked two congressional investigations of the FDA's acceptance of fraudulent safety data," including "complete fabrication of patient enrollment" and "inappropriate trial methods, when it reviewed the drug for approval" (Ross, 2007, p. 1601). Both cases serve as an indication of the reasons why the postapproval process is increasingly important to study as well as the process that pharmaceuticals undergo in order to be withdrawn from market. The decade of the 1990s saw evolution and change in the pharmaceutical approval systems of many industrialized countries (Rawson & Kaitin, 2003). In both Canada and the United States, "a focal point of the changes was to ensure that the review and approval process did not delay patients' access to important new" pharmaceuticals (Rawson & Kaitin, 2003, p. 1403). In addition, research on regulatory outcomes regarding pharmaceuticals became concerned with the "pharmaceutical lag" thesis, the claim that many pharmaceuticals are not approved as quickly in some countries. Building on this thesis, researchers have focused on whether regulations have "hampered industrial innovation or denied doctors' significant therapies for their patients" (Abraham & Davis, 2005, p. 882; Epstein, 1996; Lexchin, 2006a; Rawson & Kaitin, 2003). Conversely, little attention has been paid to the other aspect of the pharmaceutical lag thesis—that of mandatory pharmaceutical withdrawals, which is one that is inherently important to understanding the benefits and limitations of a proapproval regulatory process (Abraham & Davis, 2005). By focusing on two case studies, this book will undertake a systematic comparative analysis of the differing regulatory processes concerned with bringing about pharmaceutical withdrawals in Canada and the United States.

"Although reasons and circumstances" for the withdrawal of pharmaceuticals vary, the "trigger for discontinuation is most often new information becoming available that changes the risk–benefit evaluation from one favoring benefit to one in which risk predominates" (Rawson & Kaitin, 2003, p. 1406). Very often, these risks present themselves as serious adverse reactions. Even when well documented, however, proven serious side effects rarely induce governing bodies to withdraw pharmaceutical products immediately, as the side effects are often contested and questioned (e.g., Food and Drug Administration, 2005a). Moreover, the governing bodies' decisions can vary nationally. Considering the global society that we live in, along with major modes of international communication, not to mention the fact that scientific and medical information is shared and transferred worldwide almost instantaneously, one would suppose that developed nations especially would be very well coordinated and synchronized in terms of withdrawing pharmaceuticals off of the market. However, temporal variations between the FDA in the United States and Health Canada range up to 14 years in length (Department of Health and Human Services, 1998b; Rawson & Kaitin, 2003). The 14-year gap is the longest on record and was evidenced by two separate pharmaceuticals—the pain-reliever dipyrone and the anticancer pharmaceutical, urethane, both of which were first withdrawn in Canada in 1963, then later in the United States in 1977. More recent withdrawals, although not involving as variable a length of time, nonetheless span years, including the withdrawal of the muscle relaxant chlormezanone (1991 in Canada and 1996 in the United States) and the gastrointestinal pharmaceutical cisapride (1995 in the United States and 2000 in Canada). In addition, occasionally a pharmaceutical's unfavorable risk-to-benefit ratio has led to its withdrawal in one country, while the other country instead opts for changes to its prescribing information, or chooses to continue sales nonetheless. My research will therefore concentrate on side effects as key factors in operationalizing pharmaceutical safety hazards and will explore why such large discrepancies in time and mode of action exist between the two federal departments in ordering pharmaceutical withdrawals. Undoubtedly, such understanding is vital in making "rational judgments about the public health protective performance of regulation" as well as in providing critical insight into the appropriateness of subsequent policy shifts and direction (Abraham & Davis, 2005, p. 882).

I will be situating my examination of the scientific, institutional, and sociopolitical factors influencing and influenced by pharmaceutical withdrawals in two pharmaceutical compound case studies: pemoline (Cylert®) and tolcapone (Tasmar®). Pemoline, a central nervous system stimulant used for the treatment of attention deficit hyperactivity disorder (ADHD), was first approved for use in 1975 in the United States. Between its 1975 approval and 1996, there were 193 adverse reactions involving the liver reported to the FDA, all of which involved youths under the age of 20. In addition to having no demonstrated unique therapeutic benefit over other ADHD pharmaceuticals introduced earlier, the pharmaceutical was known to have caused at least 21 cases of liver failure, including 13 resulting in liver transplantation or death, as of 1996. The pharmaceutical's unfavorable risk-to-benefit ratio led to its withdrawal in Canada in 1999, while the FDA opted for two separate changes to the pemoline label, in 1996 and 1999, before completely withdrawing the pharmaceutical in 2005 (Hogan, 2000; Lexchin, 2005). The other pharmaceutical studied, tolcapone, was approved in both Canada and the United States in late 1997 as a treatment for management of severe movement abnormalities associated with Parkinson's disease. Based on reports of two tolcapone-related deaths outside Canada, and one in Canada, Health Canada immediately suspended all sales of the pharmaceutical within one year of its approval (Health Canada Advisory, 1998). In the United States, however, tolcapone remains on the market, albeit with added warnings regarding possible liver damage.

The two pharmaceuticals in question serve as examples illustrating broader social and scientific phenomena occurring in the fields of science and medicine. Actor network theory (ANT) is a distinctive approach to social theory and research concerned with the processes by which scientific disputes become closed, ideas accepted, and tools and methods adopted—that is, with how decisions are made about what is known (Latour, 2005). According to the model, the work of science consists of the enrollment and juxtaposition of heterogeneous "actors"—researchers, journal articles, funders, grants, papers at scientific conferences, and so on—which need continual management. An actor network, then, is the issue being studied as it is linked together with all of these influencing actors, which again are linked, producing a network.

CHAPTER 1

ACTOR NETWORK THEORY

The image is beautiful: just as glands secrete hormones, laboratories secrete reality.

—John Law and Mol (1995, p. 291)

"In the early 1980s Bruno Latour and Michel Callon at the École des Mines in Paris developed actor network theory (ANT)" with the goal of "explaining complex networks in scientific research settings" through a social theory adjusted to science and technology studies (Callon & Latour, 1981; Williams-Jones & Graham, 2003, p. 272). A branch of science and technology studies (Hess, 1997), ANT "shares the conviction that greater critical attention and empirical study should be directed at the practice of science" (Williams-Jones & Graham, 2003, p. 272). As opposed to earlier social scientific studies of sciences that focused on the laboratory setting (Latour, 1987; Latour & Woolgar, 1979), "more recent ANT analyses include investigations of science and technology development outside the laboratory and in the public and private sectors" (e.g., de Laet & Mol, 2000; John Law & Callon, 1992; Williams-Jones & Graham, 2003, p. 272).

More specifically, ANT is interested in uncovering and unraveling, but not necessarily explaining, the multiplicities of what we, as members of the general public, generally take for granted regarding medicine, science, and their emanated facts. This is accomplished by thorough description and by the following and recording of practices and individuals, as well as institutions and objects, through their actions and doings. The object in question—such as disease or a pharmaceutical—tends to vary from one practice to another simply because it is seen a little differently by each of those who work with it and encounter it. These histories and viewpoints of those around it cause the object's reality to multiply theoretically. For example, in Mol's ethnography of atherosclerosis[1] in *The Body Multiple*, she examined the daily diagnosis and treatment of the disease. From one moment, place, machine, specialty, or treatment to the next, a slightly varied version of the disease is discussed, measured, observed, and treated, depending on the history, interests, and profession of the actors (Mol, 2002). As Mol (p. 5) wrote, "The body, the patient, the disease, the doctor, the technician, the technology; all of these are more than one, more than singular." These multiple views do not, however, imply fragmentation, but rather a multiplicity of arteriosclerosis. This begs the question of how these multiple views of actors are related, since even if actors differ from one practice to another, there are relations between these practices. The answer lies in the fact that "necessarily falling into fragments, multiple objects tend to hang together" through intertwined histories of knowledge, power, science, and society (Mol, pp. 5, 62). Consequently, according to Latour (1987, p. 12), "[W]hen things hold [together], they start becoming true." Attending to the multiplicity of reality opens up the possibility of studying this extraordinary achievement and in the process, answering important questions about substantive topics.

"The great advantage of following scientific facts is that as the name indicates, they are fabricated; they exist in many different shapes and at very different stages of completion" (Latour, 2005, p. 118). While all these differences and tribulations were hidden when they were used as the "elementary building blocks" of "the world," they provide massive amounts of information as soon as they are brought back into their "factories," namely their laboratories and research institutes, when a pharmaceutical is considered for withdrawal (Latour, 2005, p. 118). The sites of ANT's interest are no longer limited to laboratories, however. The prevalence of settings in which science and technology are found and can be studied today is, indeed, the great virtue of contemporary science and technology. In fact, as Latour (2005, p. 119) wrote, "[I]t has extended itself so much, in so many settings, in ever closer intimacy with daily life and ordinary concerns, that it is hard to follow a course of action anywhere in industrial societies without bumping into one of [ANT's] outcomes." The more science and technology extend, the more they render social ties physically traceable.

ANT now offers many tools to follow facts in the making while also presenting locations and situations where they have not yet become common, taken-for-granted matters of fact (Latour, 2005). When employing ANT, it is of utmost importance that when actors and "their stories" are introduced, they are "never presented simply as matters of fact, but always as matters of concern," with their histories of creation clearly visible

(Latour, p. 120). In doing so, one discovers what was previously missing from the stories and analyses, and through this, things that seemed unanswered or inadequately explained/understood arise and can be answered.

There are other researchers who have tackled similar questions based on similar subjects with different theories. What are the strengths of ANT? For one, ANT does not disregard antagonism, struggle, and change, but rather focuses on them. This cannot be said for theories based on functionalism, for example (Mol, 2002). In 1981 Allan Young wrote the critical article entitled "When Rational Men Fall Sick: An Inquiry Into Some Assumptions Made by Medical Anthropologists." According to Mol, in it Young argued that sick people are not "rational men" as many assume, but rather "real people," while at the same time taking for granted that doctors are "rational." He believed them to be "operational" thinkers (Mol, p. 317). However, it may well be, as Mol asserted, that "doctors are as nonlinear, complex and self-contradictory as anyone else" (p. 14). In agreement with Mol, it is important to consider that doctors (or anyone in a position of authority) are strategical players playing a role—and not a role necessarily conducive to the greater good of society. In employing ANT for research, it is imperative to question what was considered fact at one time. Just like Young's assumption that doctors are naturally objective and rational, there are other presuppositions, most often found in the realm of science, waiting to be examined. In the case of pharmaceutical approval and withdrawal, one must ask these critical questions of reviewers and scientists. For instance, as they pour over submissions, are they truly unbiased and rational in their decision-making? Just because Health Canada states that reviewers objectively analyze every document submitted by manufacturers, who themselves are made to appear objective in their submissions, one cannot assume this to be true when analyzing reviewers' and manufacturers' documents for pharmaceutical approval.

1.1. EXAMINING THE IMPORTANCE OF ACTORS

According to ANT, "[E]ntities, whether people or technologies, are not static and do not have significance in and of themselves. Instead, they achieve significance through relations with other entities," and "if differences exist, it is because they are generated in the relations that produce them. Not because they exist, as it were, in the order of things" (John Law, 2001, as cited in Williams-Jones & Graham, 2003, p. 272). In effect, individual people and things become important only when, and because, they are a part of relationships with others. According to Singleton and Michael (1993, as cited in Williams-Jones & Graham, 2003, p. 272), "[I]ndividual actors are considered to be ambivalent or ambiguous...not static or unitary; they will change over time, across social and political contexts, and in their relations with other actors." It is only in aggregates that these individuals become important and available for study, at least according to ANT.

Both humans and nonhumans—such as the pharmaceuticals in question—and scientific reports and documents "are treated as epistemologically equivalent for the purpose of critical analysis and are considered to be actors, inasmuch as they have the ability to act and to be acted upon" (Williams-Jones & Graham, 2003, p. 272), and contain "embedded knowledges" (Mol, 2002, p. 15). As Mol (p. 48) wrote, "[T]he knowledge incorporated in practices does not reside in subjects alone, but also in buildings, knives, dyes and desks." The authority and influence of a human actor is generally seen as being self-explanatory and noncontroversial, "although it can become an issue when an individual's independence is constrained by mental illness or by differential power relations in the form of class or gender" (Williams-Jones & Graham, 2003, p. 272). Taking into account objects, technologies, and inhuman entities, such as corporations, and assigning them the "human" qualities of action and power may appear nonsensical at first. As Williams-Jones and Graham noted, however,

> [e]xamination of object-human interactions demonstrates that objects and other non-human entities do affect human behaviour. For example, a telephone may appear to be an ordinary, passive technology, but this impression changes when the telephone rings. Even if one decides to ignore the noise, the telephone has still provoked a decision making process and elicited a non-response. (2003, p. 272)

Furthermore, Mol asserted that "[i]f pulled and pushed a bit, [the social sciences] may be broadened to encompass subject/objects of all kinds" (2002, p. 34). ANT is the result of this broadening: Actors in the form of objects, such as pharmaceuticals for example, influence, heal, hurt, kill, save—in short, they *do* things. Why not study them at parity with physical subjects?

Latour wrote about nonhuman actors in the following way:

> ANT is not the empty claim that objects do things "instead" of human actors: it simply says that no science of the social can even begin if the question of who and what participates in the action is not first of all thoroughly explored, even though it might mean letting elements in which, for lack of a better term, we would call non humans…The project of ANT is simply to extend the list and modify the shapes and figures of those assembled as participants and to design a way to make them act as a durable whole. (Latour, 2005, p. 72)

Following along the same lines, when working with ANT, it is necessary to accept that the continuity of any course of action will rarely solely consist of human-to-human connections or of object-to-object ones, but will most likely "zigzag from one to the other" in constructing a scene wherein humans and nonhumans are fused together (Latour, 2005, p. 75). According to Latour (1993), both human and nonhuman actors are "necessarily heterogeneous and have varying degrees of commitment, skill, prejudice, and constraints associated with them; they are often hybrids of the 'social,' 'technical' and 'personal'" (as cited in Williams-Jones & Graham, 2003, p. 273). At the technical level, a chemical entity may be involved in biochemical assays or in pioneering clinical trials. The validity and reliability of the compound is "determined and disputed by scientists, clinicians, and epidemiologists, and there may be better or worse treatments or others yet to be discovered" for the same condition (Williams-Jones & Graham, 2003, p. 273). Access by patients to the compound and its corresponding treatment regime "may be restricted to certain individuals based on professional standards in the medical community, which may nevertheless vary geographically" (Williams-Jones & Graham, 2003, p. 273; see also Gomart, 2002). This brings into effect both social and technical actors in the form of professional codes of ethics and standards embodied by medical professionals and their relation to, and impact on, patients who comprise the personal or social, especially if these patients are assembled into associations such as patient support groups. In order to understand "how these relations create meaning and to describe the various actors" (e.g., the condition, compound, "patients, technicians, patent owners, clinicians, scientists, the general public, and policy makers), it is useful to think in terms of networks of relations, or more specifically, actor networks" (Williams-Jones & Graham, 2003, p. 273).

1.2. Actors Form Actor Networks

Pharmaceutical prescription and use as a procedure is clearly and undoubtedly composed of many entities, both human and nonhuman, which interact in order to form one undifferentiated arrangement held together by a set of connections. The word *network* describes such resources concentrated in a few places comprising knots and nodes and being connected with one another through links and "mesh." These connections, whether physical or virtual, transform the "scattered resources" into a net that may seem to extend everywhere (Latour, 1987, p. 180). However, being connected, being interconnected, or being heterogeneous is not enough. It all depends on the sort of action that is flowing from one to the other—hence the words *net* and *work*. As Latour wrote, "Really, we should say 'worknet' instead of 'network'. It is the work and the movement, the flow, and the changes that should be stressed" (2005, p. 143). When speaking of a pharmaceutical, the scientist, physician, or patient does not claim "the therapeutic value of a medication, of an isolated substance; instead, they describe the medical benefit of a treatment. In doing so, they shift from an isolated substance to the description of a heterogeneous network of practices" (Gomart, 2002, p. 106). It is with mapping these associations and the worknet that emerges between them that this study is concerned. For example, when a patient is said to be undergoing cancer treatment, they may be undergoing surgery, radiation therapy, pharmaceutical administration, or chemotherapy. Sometimes one type of treatment is used, while at other times, a combination of treatments may be used. Patients and families may also hear the term *investigational treatment* (British Columbia Cancer Agency, 2008). This means that the treatment is being studied in a clinical trial with the help of researchers, laboratories and their technicians, academic institutions, and the manufacturers themselves. Furthermore, support programs, alternative therapies, or complementary programs may also be employed, and all are referred to as aspects of "the treatment" (British Columbia Cancer Agency, 2008).

Williams-Jones and Graham (2003, p. 273) characterized actor networks as "shifting systems of alliances 'performed' into existence by the actors involved" and automatically "including both human and non-human elements." They added that networks are "inherently unstable over time (ambivalent), have to be continually maintained through engagements (enrollment) of the actors involved, and may fail and be replaced by other networks" (p. 273). In short, there is nothing static, stable, or permanent about any one network. Neither is there any one central actor or ultimate source of power over the grouping of actors. In the case of pharmaceuticals, it may be that the actual compound may appear to be at the center of the network and by extension, "hold ultimate power" in it. However, if that pharmaceutical ceases to adequately "work," be approved, or be believed in or if it is withdrawn from the market, it will no longer serve as a focal point. At that time, the other actors may search for, work with, or become actors involved in another network centered on another pharmaceutical. Clearly, there are many different entities and many different ways of viewing power in the network:

> If we wish to know the origins of power and structure in a network, that is, what drives the network or brings it into being, then we need to consider all the components that collaborate, cooperate, compete and lead to proliferation, persistence or perishing of that network, in effect the multiplicity of the pharmaceutical. (Williams-Jones & Graham, 2003)

The challenge of ANT, then, is to open up and better understand the underlying progressions and elements of the actors in the networks, all of whom may not be readily apparent (Williams-Jones & Graham, 2003). A good text "elicits the networks of actors when it allows the writer to trace a set of relations" in order to tell their combined, heterogeneous story (Latour, 2005, p. 129).

According to Williams-Jones and Graham (2003), in order to start following actor interactions, it is necessary to develop a preliminary sketch of the network in question by tracing each actor's many social connections. Figure 1 maps some of the central actors involved in the development of the pharmaceuticals in question. Undoubtedly, this task is complicated by actors participating in, or "being enrolled" in, many networks that may or may not overlap with the network under investigation (Latour, 2005, p. 29). One may think of an actor network as expanding or contracting infinitely, with each actor comprising a node in another network (Latour). Given this density, separating "foreground" from "background" becomes difficult (Williams-Jones & Graham, 2003), since every piece of information, and more specifically each additional actor no matter how insignificant they may appear, "will provide the analyst with a bewildering array of entities to account for the how's and whys [*sic*] of any course of action" (Latour, p. 47).

The challenge of simplifying actor networks has been addressed by the idea of creating "black boxes" (Akrich, 1992, as cited in Williams-Jones & Graham, 2003). "As networks become stronger and more stable, they can, for the purpose of analysis by ANT researchers, be regarded as points or nodes in a larger network," in which case "the supporting network is black boxed." In figure 1, each of the actors could also be expanded in order to "produce its own complex network" (Williams-Jones & Graham, 2003, p. 274), as is illustrated in the attached boxes for the Public Health Care Services and Treatment Compound nodes. The Public Health Care Services box can be expanded to include its own network comprised of health care professionals, physical settings, physical treatments, and associated, yet very important, actors such as Medicare and budgetary aspects. Similarly, the Treatment

FIGURE 1. Network of a health disorder.

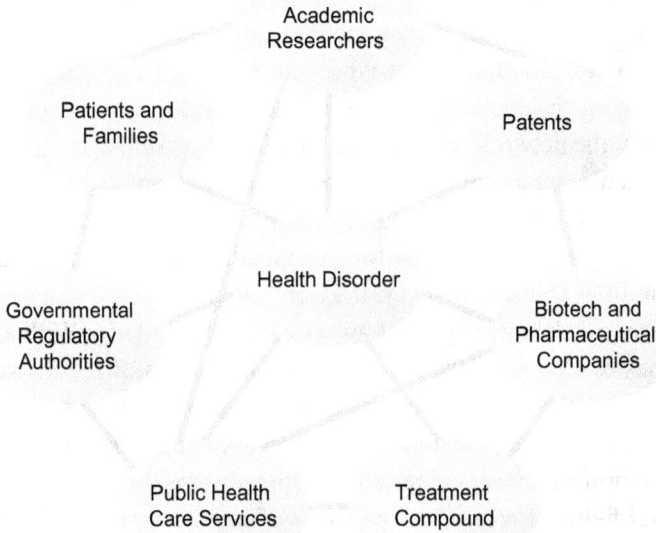

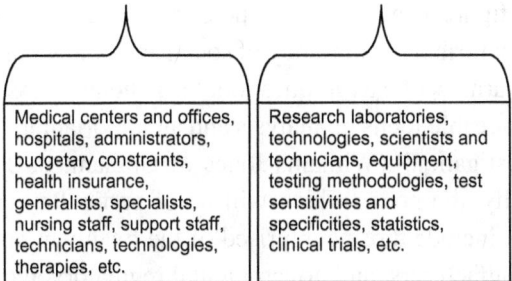

Academic
Researchers

Patients and
Families

Patents

Health Disorder

Governmental
Regulatory
Authorities

Biotech and
Pharmaceutical
Companies

Public Health
Care Services

Treatment
Compound

Medical centers and offices, hospitals, administrators, budgetary constraints, health insurance, generalists, specialists, nursing staff, support staff, technicians, technologies, therapies, etc.

Research laboratories, technologies, scientists and technicians, equipment, testing methodologies, test sensitivities and specificities, statistics, clinical trials, etc.

Source. Schematic adapted from Williams-Jones and Graham (2003, p. 274).

Compound node can be expanded to include its network of pharmaceutical-related characteristics, actors, and sites. These include the drug's sensitivity, specificity, and predicted value in treating a condition; testing methods; evidence-based medicine; laboratories; and all those who determine and influence these, including technicians. As can be seen from the two expanded nodes, the networks of each are not mutually exclusive.

Such compartmentalization of actors does not reduce a network to an essential capturing of the whole; indeed, it is the "partial connections that allow for the diasporic translations and pluralities that acknowledge the uncertainties of ANT, and which are most celebrated" (John Law, 1999, p. 10, as cited in Williams-Jones & Graham, 2003, p. 274). The intricacies of the network remain, although for purposes of analysis, they can be moved to the "background," and allow the network to appear as if its current form was never contested or disputed. As is the case for many other fields of research, "the focus of inquiry drives the choice of the most appropriate scale of analysis" (Williams-Jones & Graham, 2003, p. 274). Furthermore, "[w]hile the network illustrated in figure 1 may be only one of many networks that could usefully contribute to the study of social and policy implications" of the pharmaceuticals in question, "it is nonetheless a discrete and manageable focus of analysis and an important locus for further investigation" (Williams-Jones & Graham, p. 275). More specifically, the nodes which will be of particular centrality to this book include those comprised of the treatment compounds, their manufacturers, and governmental regulatory agencies, and the individuals providing public health care services—most specifically, physicians and by extension, their patients. This is due to the fact that the actors in these specific nodes emerged to be of utmost importance and sources of the most "action" in my research on the two pharmaceuticals' approval and withdrawal histories in Canada and the United States. It is imperative to remember, however, that another researcher or a slight change in topic could easily result in a focus on different nodes.

1.3. TRANSLATION

Each actor in a network is largely independent and free to either resist or accommodate other actors and their influences. As a result, one can surmise that there must be some "glue" that encourages each actor to maintain involvement in a network (Williams-Jones & Graham, 2003, p. 275). This glue is "translation" (Callon, 1986, p. 202). Key to translation is that each actor, whether composed of an individual or an assembly, is assumed to possess individual interests. In ANT, a network's stability is seen as resulting from this continual translation of interests between actors. In human-to-human interactions, translation is equivalent to the negotiation of common interests; in human and nonhuman interactions, inter-action is accomplished through the creation of scripts (discussed in the following text; Williams-Jones & Graham). "Policies, behaviors, motivations, and goals are translated from one actor to another; and actors are themselves translated and changed in their interactions with others" (Callon, as cited in Williams-Jones & Graham, p. 275).

As has been noted by previous ANT researchers, the development of technologies is also "inherently a process of translation" (Williams-Jones & Graham, 2003, p. 276). As the technological device passes through the stages of design, manufacture, marketing, and use, it will undoubtedly and necessarily change. It has been stated that

> technologies are not simply passive and are never value-neutral, but however, always exist in value-laden social and technical relations. During the design phase, objects have embedded within them a "script" or set of instructions that

> determine how the technology will function and the extent to which it may be shaped by other actors. Technical and normative values built into the technology, and its supporting documents, marketing, etc., attempt to prescribe specific patterns of use while restricting others. (Prout, 1996, as cited in Williams-Jones & Graham, 2003, p. 276)

The development and use of pharmaceuticals also has a story and a larger social context that continues to influence each actor network in the larger health care setting long after initial approval for widespread use. Technology, such as that embodied by pharmaceuticals, composes an important aspect of the worknet of medicine. It can be said that human makers can be "seen" in machines and implements, as well as in their work; both are disguised under the guise of technology (Latour, 1999). As such, it is important to "restore the human labour that stands behind those idols," as it, too, leads to further actors in this field—the makers (Latour, 1999). As Latour wrote,

> [W]e hourly encounter hundreds, even thousands, of absent makers who are remote in time and space yet simultaneously active and present...we rely on many delegated actions that themselves make us do things on behalf of others who are no longer here. (1994, p. 40)

In order to understand technological advancement and expansion, it is necessary to "move beyond a linear model of technology diffusion or transfer. In fact, a simple binary model of technological-push and market-pull is insufficient" (Williams-Jones & Graham, 2003, p. 277). Furthermore,

> [t]he complex interaction between the social and the technological often renders the two inseparable. In implementing a new technology, it may be necessary to "allow"

it to drift into unexpected situations; if the technology is going to "work," it must be open to change. Innovations configure the user, defining who may use it and how, but they also modify existing social structures and create new ones. (Williams-Jones & Graham, 2003, p. 277)

This could not be truer of both pemoline and tolcapone, which drifted into new off-label uses, as well as more restricted roles due to adverse reactions as time wore on.

1.4. THE EXAMINATION OF BLACK BOXES

ANT is an approach that involves curiosity about describing and analyzing tensions between actors, networks, and technologies and how they are displayed in daily life (Latour, 1996; John Law, 1999). Any translation of a network or technology may be unsuccessful (or succeed in unexpected ways), and it is in these failures that embedded standards and principles are often best revealed (Holmstrom & Stalder, 2001; John Law & Callon, 1992, as cited in Williams-Jones & Graham, 2003, p. 277). In fact, "controversies provide the analyst with an essential resource to render the social connections traceable" (Latour, 2005, p. 30). Important insights that enable comprehensive ethical analysis and social critique include the following: (a) Science can be seen as inextricably linked to politics, (b) human and nonhuman actors are necessary parts of networks, (c) and technologies are inherently value laden. ANT can be used for a strictly function-alist analysis, but it can also be used as a way of undermining the functionalist and determinist models of network building (John Law, 1999). Thus, while ANT does not explicitly include critical analysis of institutions, technologies, or actors, such analysis is not impeded but, rather, is important to consider when studying topics such as pharmaceutical withdrawal.

Latour's concept of a "black box" applies to this area of study in the following manner: When a pharmaceutical is approved for sale, it is assumed to do its task of remedying maladies safely and effectively, and as such, it is black boxed and left to do its work. Any controversies surrounding the drug's approval or use are silenced, or at least have great difficulty gaining attention. The withdrawal process is one of slowly prying open the box until it no longer holds together and eventually ceases to exist. The dismantling of the initial approval process is, in fact, failure for the black boxes known as facts to hold. By employing ANT, this book uncovers and explores the networks of actors and the kinds of evidence and data that they enrolled in generating final conclusions about two pharmaceuticals and how these conclusions varied between the United States and Canada. The idea that "facts" about pharmaceutical safety are so differently interpreted and used in the two countries makes this study an important wedge into understanding how knowledge is brokered in the contemporary market for pharmaceuticals.

In the field of pharmaceuticals, it is precisely when functionalist models of analysis fail, as in when networks and black boxes "fall apart" in regard to the continued approval of a pharmaceutical, that critical analysis of the various actors involved can lead to improved understanding of what kept the boxes "intact" initially and why certain assumptions, norms, and values did not "hold" in order to keep the box closed perpetually. As a result, ANT provides us with a method for attending to the various ways in which differences are handled in various sites and situations, an effective framework with which to understand discrepant pharmaceutical regulatory processes in a sociohistorical context, and a way of wondering "when and where we might do better" (Mol, 2002, p. 116).

ENDNOTE

1. Atherosclerosis is a gradual obstruction of the arteries, particularly those of the legs.

CHAPTER 2

METHODS

It is only by constantly comparing complex repertoires
of action that sociologists may become able to register
data—a task that seems always very hard for the sociolo-
gists of the social who have to filter out everything which
does not look in advance like a uniformed "social actor."
Recording *not filtering out,* describing *not disciplining,*
these are the Laws and the Prophets.

—Latour (2005, p. 55, emphasis in original)

As mentioned previously, actor network theory (ANT) may be conceptualized as both a theory and a methodology. As Latour wrote, ANT does not tell us things about the world, as in how the social world is, but rather suggests *how* to study things (Latour, 2004, as cited in Kaplan, Truex, Wastell, Wood-Harper, & DeGross, 2004, p. 265, italics in original). So what does ANT say about conducting an empirical study? Its advice is simple in that following the actors through whichever means are most relevant and useful is a keystone of the entire method. It is only through the following of actors that one can deduce information on their worknets of action and interaction, and through this, one can deduce information about black boxes, facts, and these facts' formations and failures (Klecun, 2004). As was examined previously, this entails the dismissal of preconceived expectations or theories about actors and networks as guides for research. For example, one should not make distinctions "between the size of actors, between the real and the unreal, between what is necessary and what is contingent, between the technical and social" (Callon & Latour, 1981, p. 291, as cited in Klecun, 2004, p. 265). According to Latour (2004, p. 65), "[A]ctors themselves make everything, including their own frames, their own theories, their own contexts, their own metaphysics, even their own ontologies." "Thus, in commenting on how to write research findings, he told us not to impose our own frameworks or concepts but just to describe" (Klecun, 2004, p. 265). It is the loaded description that provides insights into the situation.

Klecun asked, "Is there anything more to the methodology of ANT?" (2004, p. 266). No and yes. No, because there are no specific outlines or structures to follow when proceeding along with an ANT-based study. Yes, because ANT does provide us with certain helpful suggestions to consult and employ when conducting research. For example, "ANT elaborates on the processes of construction and deconstruction of actor networks in terms of translation" (Callon, 1986, as cited in Klecun, 2004, p. 265). It also describes which approaches are useful in order to discover and describe actors, their involvement in assemblies, and their actions.

Methodologically, ANT has two major approaches: one being the examination of documents and texts, the other, "following the actor," wherein the actor is not necessarily a human participant.

Aspects of both were performed in collecting evidence for this book. First, archival research was performed on records of meetings of subcommittees considering the pharmaceuticals of interest first for approval and subsequently for withdrawal. The Therapeutic Products Programme at Health Canada conducts risk–benefit assessments of treatments in Canada, as does the Center for Biologics Evaluation and Research division of the Food and Drug Administration (FDA) in the United States. Records of deliberations for both of the pharmaceuticals in question, as well as certain supporting documents employed by both subcommittees, are archived on the Internet and when unavailable, were requested in hardcopy under Freedom of Information Acts in both countries. Those from the FDA were promptly sent, while those from Health Canada have yet to arrive. These "reviewer documents" were comprised of new drug applications, pharmacology reviews, chemical reviews, environmental reviews, bioavailability reviews, clinical reviews, adverse reaction reviews, product monographs, memorandums, and approval letters on both pharmaceuticals. In addition, letters from the FDA and Health Canada to manufacturers were also analyzed when access to them was possible. Regarding pharmaceutical withdrawal, withdrawal petitions, memorandums, committee reviews, "Dear Health Care Provider" letters, and press releases were analyzed. Lastly, documents regarding how Health Canada and the FDA weigh risks and benefits were analyzed.

All relevant scientific literature, publications by the regulatory agencies, pharmaceutical trade press publications—such as *Scrip*—and media reports from relevant time periods were also analyzed in order to uncover how each pharmaceutical was depicted when it was first approved and then again when it was withdrawn. The time span analyzed ranged from the first mention of each drug in the scientific and clinical literature to the time when each drug was withdrawn. The great majority of publications occurred during the time of approval and again during the time of withdrawal. I examined whether there was a difference in the type of media coverage during each time period, as well as how these pharmaceuticals were studied and framed in the research literature.

In order to determine the overall tone of journal articles on both pemoline and tolcapone prior to approval and onwards, a database containing journal articles from relevant time periods was constructed for each pharmaceutical. Medline, an electronic search engine which indexes articles from 1966 onward, was used as the main source of data on articles and authors relating to pemoline and tolcapone publishing. The database was first searched using the search term *pemoline.ti*, which identified articles in which pemoline was featured in the title. The search was also limited to *human* and *journal article*, resulting in a set of 143 articles. The data set was downloaded and imported into a Microsoft® Excel® spreadsheet. This comprised the pemoline database. An identical procedure was followed for the search term *tolcapone.ti*, resulting in a set of 89 articles. Each article in each database was analyzed and categorized regarding its overall tone, whether supportive, critical, or neutral towards the pharmaceutical in question. Each article's tone was classified largely on authors' conclusions concerning the drug in question in regard to safety, efficacy, and overall medical merit. Supportive conclusions most often referred to the drug as "well-tolerated," "recommended for use," or "current adverse reaction reports are overestimated." Critical conclusions included statements such as "not currently suitable for administration," "clear limitations in efficacy," and "induced serious adverse reactions such as..." Neutral conclusions were most often linked to the structure of the journal article, wherein it served as a biochemical, rather than clinical, purpose. Biochemical articles dealt with the physical properties of the compound rather than its treatment outcomes, and as such, did not offer a conclusion regarding the drug's treatment. Otherwise, neutrality was determined when authors claimed that, indeed, the drug offered no significant advantage over other treatments for the condition in question, and as such, these articles were not supportive or critical in tone.

This database was also supplemented with a cited reference search of Web of Science, formerly known as the Science Citation Index. This tool is a multidisciplinary index to the journal literature of the sciences. It fully indexes 5,900 major journals across 150 scientific disciplines, while also including all cited references captured from indexed articles. A search of all articles published in the Web of Science with *pemoline* in the title and not limited by language or article type resulted in 288 articles. Using these articles, a cross-tabulation was created to indicate the 10 most cited articles. These articles were then examined for evidence of manufacturers' involvement or support in the research. The same procedure was then followed for tolcapone, with a result of 166 articles.

In the preceding sections, three concepts—actors, actor networks, and translation—were briefly explored in order to illustrate how they might contribute to an understanding of the various interactions between individuals, organizations, and technology. The following chapters will serve as the focal points describing what is occurring in the actor networks of pemoline and tolcapone, specifically those facets which led to the technologies being developed, integrated, and later withdrawn from market(s) as part of public health care in Canada and the United States. Tracing the path of these technological actors highlights the numerous, complex social and ethical issues associated with approving and withdrawing pharmaceuticals from the market.

In addition, through the method of tracing of assemblies and practices, "space" is left open for unexpected actors to emerge. This is precisely the goal of ANT—practices are not always as objective and straightforward as they appear, and through their tracing, some previously unthought of, yet important, actors may surface.

A central feature of ANT is "letting the actors speak for themselves" by allowing their "life stories" to come to the forefront, unaided by prescribed theories and analyses. This was done in my study because the main indicator of quality for an ANT account is when "the actors are allowed to be stronger than the analyst" rather than the analyst "doing all of the talking" (Latour, 2005, p. 30). Actors are always engaged in the business of "mapping the social context in which they are placed," and as such, they "do the sociology for the sociologists and sociologists learn from the actors what makes up their set of associations" (Latour, p. 32). It is for this reason that the main actors involved (identified in the following text), as well as their enrollment in controversies in approving, monitoring, using, and withdrawing pharmaceuticals, are paramount to analyzing each pharmaceutical's lifespan.

By acquainting myself with these central actors and their enrollment in networks and controversies, it became more and more apparent what context each pharmaceutical was introduced into, as well as why further events unfolded as they did. In doing so, the actors began to speak for themselves and increasingly make apparent why their "life stories" turned out as they did. Through this process, the final conclusions about the two pharmaceuticals, and how these conclusions varied between the United States and Canada, become apparent. It is for this specific reason that the method of organizing this book was chosen: The actors, followed by their enrollment in a network, are allowed to expose "who" they are first and how they are enrolled, after which it becomes apparent to the reader how they fit into the broader universe of pharmaceutical use and regulation and why they were treated as they were. Throughout the process, I asked, "What is surprising about the stories surrounding these two pharmaceuticals and the process of their approval and withdrawal?" From there, I noted things that seemed unanswered or inadequately explained: "What might be missing from these stories and analyses?"

The main actors involved in this study include Health Canada, the FDA in the United States, the pharmaceutical industry, physicians and patients as a collective, as well as the pharmaceuticals in question. This book, therefore, begins by highlighting each of the major actors, as I gathered from my research, in detail, including a breakdown of each pharmaceutical's "lifespan" in the Description chapter. This is followed by a thorough description of the assemblies produced in order to compose the pemoline and tolcapone networks, respectively. The actors and their enrollment in collectivities termed *pemoline* or *tolcapone* are then relayed to the reader, after which a deeper examination of failures and breakdowns in the seemingly well-contrived networks is analyzed. It is important to note, however, that some unexpected actors emerged during the course of my research, particularly in preparing the description. These actors are first described and then included in the Analysis chapter along with the major actors highlighted previously. Through these steps, it becomes evident why, in fact, the regulatory processes concerned with effectuating pharmaceutical withdrawals in Canada and the United States "treated" pemoline and tolcapone so differently and what can be learned from this examination of the two pharmaceuticals' histories.

CHAPTER 3

DESCRIPTION

3.1. THE DRUG APPROVAL PROCESS OF HEALTH CANADA

Prescription pharmaceuticals, vitamins, and vaccines play an important role in helping Canadians to live healthy lives. As a result, more than 22,000 of such pharmaceutical products are available in Canada today, all of which have passed Health Canada's safety standards (Health Canada, 2006b).

New pharmaceutical products are approved for sale in Canada once they have successfully passed a review process assessing their effectiveness at treating prescribed conditions safely. Responsibility for this review process rests with Health Canada's Health Products and Food Branch (HPFB), which in theory, assesses each pharmaceutical without bias, based purely on scientific and medical merit, by subjecting it to a series of steps.

Before a therapeutic product is authorized for sale in Canada, the manufacturer must provide HPFB with "scientific evidence of its safety, efficacy and quality, as defined by regulations" by filing a new pharmaceutical submission (Kelly, Lazzaro, & Petersen, 2007, S5). A new pharmaceutical submission, which "typically involves hundreds of volumes of data," contains information from the manufacturer regarding animal tests, chemistry, and manufacturing data, as well as results from clinical trials of various phases (Kelly et al., 2007, S5). It is the role of regulatory pharmaceutical submission evaluators in Canada to critically assess both the data submitted and the manufacturer's (referred to as "sponsor" by both Health Canada and the FDA), interpretation of the data in order to reach an evidence-, and context-based recommendation as to the potential benefits and potential harms associated with taking the pharmaceutical.

According to Marra, Lynd, Anis, and Esdaile (2006), "[c]linical trials are classified into three sequential phases: Phase 1, safety studies; Phase 2, small scale efficacy and dose-finding studies; and Phase 3, studies that examine the outcomes (safety and efficacy) of pharmaceuticals in larger groups of patients over longer periods of time" (p. 9). Phase 1 trials generally involve testing the pharmaceutical in "small samples of either healthy or diseased individuals for a short period of time to provide initial data on appropriate dosing and common adverse events" (Marra et al., p. 9). In Phase 2 trials, the pharmaceutical is studied in larger samples of patients, often treated with varying dosage strengths in order to "determine the relative efficacy of the agent" (Marra et al., p. 9). Finally, Phase 3 studies "generally involve the comparison of the new pharmaceutical with either placebo or existing therapy indicated for use in the same disease state to evaluate outcomes (i.e., both safety and efficacy) over longer periods of time" (Marra et al., p. 9; see also Lipsky & Sharp, 2001; Myers

& Moore, 1987). HPFB has the authority to conduct inspections of clinical trials for pharmaceuticals and natural health products. Currently, however, only about 2% of the clinical trials conducted in Canada for pharmaceuticals are inspected annually.[1] If the clinical studies demonstrate that the potential benefits appear to outweigh the potential risks of the pharmaceutical compound, the manufacturer can file a new pharmaceutical submission with the Therapeutic Products Directorate at the HPFB (Kelly et al., 2007; Marra et al., 2006). The new pharmaceutical submission must contain all preclinical and clinical data available for the pharmaceutical in order for the agency to determine that the pharmaceutical "is safe, efficacious, that the manufacturing process is consistent with regulatory requirements, and, thus, that the final product is of high quality" (Marra et al., p. 10). In addition, "information regarding the pharmaceutical's production, source of raw materials, location of the manufacturing facilities, and packaging and labeling must also be included" (Marra et al., p. 10).

If the expected benefits of the pharmaceutical "outweigh the known potential adverse events," known as the risk–benefit equation, the HPFB will approve the pharmaceutical by "issuing a Notice of Compliance (NOC) and a Drug Identification Number (DIN)" (Marra et al., 2006, p. 10). According to Marra et al., "[T]he DIN is unique to every prescription pharmaceutical and must be printed on every container in which the pharmaceutical is packaged and marketed" (p. 10). Furthermore, the HPFB "will also review and edit the product monograph submitted by the manufacturer" (Marra et al., p. 10). For seriously debilitating conditions with few treatments, Health Canada has established a priority review process. Through this process, the HPFB can authorize a manufacturer to market a pharmaceutical before all trials are completed "under the condition that the manufacturer performs additional studies to assess the potential risks and benefits of the product" (Marra et al., p. 10; see also Kelly et al., 2007).

Once a pharmaceutical is approved for sale in Canada, the Marketed Products Directorate at Health Canada is also responsible for the postmarketing surveillance. This surveillance includes the collection and evaluation of information pertaining to adverse drug reactions and potentially acting on this information in the interest of patient safety. (Marra et al., p. 10)

3.2. THE DRUG APPROVAL PROCESS OF THE FDA

The FDA is responsible for ensuring that pharmaceuticals, as well as foods and cosmetics, are safe and effective for use by the American public. By carrying out this responsibility, the FDA monitors more than US$1 trillion worth of products, comprising US$0.25 of every US$1 spent annually by American consumers (Food and Drug Administration—Center for Drug Evaluation and Research, 2008, as cited in Lipsky & Sharp, 2001). In the 1990s alone, "more than 500 new prescription pharmaceuticals have been approved by the FDA" (Lipsky & Sharp, 2001, p. 362). Analyzing the safety and efficacy of these products is the main public health protection responsibility of the FDA, more specifically, the Center for Drug Evaluation and Research. This responsibility for pharmaceutical control involves the examination of pharmaceutical trials, preparation of products for sale, as well as monitoring the public's use of the products, including adverse reactions reports.

As in Canada, pharmaceutical development in the United States can generally be divided into phases. According to FDA requirements, a manufacturer must initially provide data indicating that the pharmaceutical is "reasonably safe for use in initial, small-scale clinical studies" (Center for Drug Evaluation and

Research, 1998, p. 5). Depending on whether the compound has been evaluated or marketed previously, the manufacturer can satisfy this requirement by compiling existing data from past laboratory or animal studies or by compiling data from previous clinical testing or marketing of the pharmaceutical in the United States or "another country whose population is relevant to the U.S. population"; additionally, the manufacturer can satisfy this requirement by beginning new studies demonstrating that the pharmaceutical is safe when administered to humans (Center for Drug Evaluation and Research, p. 5).

During preclinical pharmaceutical development, a sponsor evaluates the pharmaceutical's toxic and pharmacologic effects through laboratory and animal testing. Genotoxicity screening is performed in order to determine whether the compound affects individuals' cell DNA, and investigations are performed on absorption and metabolism, as well as on the speed with which the compound is removed from the body. At this preclinical stage, the manufacturer is required to determine the toxicity of the compound in at least two species of animals and to conduct toxicity studies ranging from 2 weeks to 3 months, depending on the proposed length of use of the compound in upcoming clinical studies (Food and Drug Administration, 1999b). After successful completion of these steps, the manufacturer can submit an application in order for the compound to be considered as an investigational new drug (IND; Center for Drug Evaluation and Research, 1998, p. 7).

When an IND is submitted to the FDA, it is assigned to one of six pharmaceutical reviewing divisions. The six pharmaceutical reviewing divisions—Chemistry, Pharmacology, Pharmacokinetics, Microbiology, Clinical, and Statistics—are responsible for specific classes of pharmaceuticals and are organizationally similar in composition. Group leaders who are medical officers serve primarily as leaders of the review team, which is loosely structured around a clinical reviewer, chemist, pharmacologist, and consumer safety officer (Myers & Moore, 1987). In addition, consultants and other support personnel, such as advisory community members from academia, are used to complement the FDA review staff when needed. Each member of the team performs his or her own review after which the review eventually becomes part of the basis for approval or nonapproval of the application. At times, the reviewers meet to "discuss issues, progress, and problems, and frequent meetings are arranged" with the manufacturer in order to discuss "certain issues or to summarize the status of the application" (Myers & Moore, p. 822). In addition, the IND must be reviewed and approved by the Institutional Review Board where the studies are to be conducted, and progress reports on clinical trials must be submitted at least annually to the FDA (Lipsky & Sharp, 2001).

If an IND is approved, the next steps are clinical Phases 1, 2, and 3, which require approximately 1, 2, and 3 years, respectively, for completion (Lipsky & Sharp, 2001). Following the completion of all three phases of clinical trials, the manufacturer analyzes all of the data and files a new drug application (NDA) containing all of the scientific information that the manufacturer has gathered to date. An NDA can also include experience with the medication from outside the United States, as well as external studies related to the pharmaceutical (Lipsky & Sharp). The NDA is then once again examined and reviewed via the same process employed for INDs.

Once the review is complete, the NDA may be either granted approval for marketing or, conversely, rejected. If the pharmaceutical is rejected, the manufacturer is provided with the reasons why in addition to information regarding reapplication for approval for the same pharmaceutical. An approval may also be conditional upon further clinical studies. For example, the FDA may request "postmarketing" or Phase 4 studies in order to further examine the pharmaceutical in another population or to perform monitoring in a specific population. Otherwise, a Phase 4 study may be instigated by the manufacturer in order to evaluate long-term effects of pharmaceutical exposure in order to determine the optimal treatment dose, to determine the pharmaceutical's effects in children, or to determine the effectiveness of the pharmaceutical for other conditions (Lipsky & Sharp, 2001).

Like Health Canada, the FDA relies solely on data that manufacturers submit to decide whether a pharmaceutical should be approved. In order to "protect the rights and welfare of people in clinical trials, and to verify the quality and integrity of data submitted," the FDA's Division of Scientific Investigations (DSI) conducts inspections of clinical investigators' study sites (Food and Drug Administration, 2005a). "FDA investigators compare information that clinical investigators provided to sponsors on case report forms with information in source documents such as medical records and lab results," wrote Carolyn Hommel, a consumer safety officer in the DSI (Food and Drug Administration, 2005a). The DSI conducts about 300 to 400 clinical investigator inspections annually. About 3% are classified in the "official action indicated" category, resulting from the observance of numerous or serious deviations from professional conduct codes, such as falsification of data.

3.3. WHAT HAPPENS ONCE A PHARMACEUTICAL IS APPROVED?

Often, many serious adverse pharmaceutical reactions are discovered only after a pharmaceutical has been on the market for years, and as such, it is therefore necessary to continue monitoring the safety and effectiveness of pharmaceuticals well after they reach the marketplace if we are to fully understand their health benefits and the potential risks associated with their use. Such "postmarket" surveillance and assessment contributes new and up-to-date information that can only be realistically acquired after a product is widely used under "real-life" conditions for a sustained period of time (Health Canada, 2006a, p. 20). In contrast to the highly structured premarketing evaluation, however, postmarketing surveillance has little structure.

Under Health Canada's Food and Pharmaceuticals Act, manufacturers are responsible for continuously reporting on the safety of their products in Canada directly to the HPFB. Manufacturers are also required to report any new information that they receive concerning serious side effects, including "any failure of the product to produce the desired effect" (Health Canada, 2006a).[2] According to the HPFB, "[T]here is a prescribed format [an adverse reaction report] and timeline for reporting adverse reactions," as well as "any studies that manufacturers have that provide new safety information" (Health Canada, p. 19). An adverse reaction report contains information about the affected patients, the suspected association between the therapeutic product and the adverse reaction, and the treatment and final outcomes of the product use. The identities of both the patient and the person reporting are kept confidential by HPFB (Health Canada). Although "patients, health professionals, manufacturers and health product regulatory authorities [are expected to] work together to monitor adverse reactions," the most common source of information about adverse reactions is voluntary reporting by health professionals and consumers (Health Canada, p. 20). Although approximately 10,000 of such adverse drug reaction reports were completed in Canada in 2004, it is commonly agreed upon that this constitutes a small fraction, or less than 10%, of all estimated adverse reactions (Lasser et al., 2002; Pirmohamed, Breckenridge, Kittering-ham, & Park, 1998; Walker & Lumley, 1987).

According to Psaty, Furberg, Ray, and Weiss, "FDA post-marketing regulations only require that pharmaceutical companies collect, review, and report to the FDA all suspected adverse drug reactions thought to be associated with the pharmaceutical in question," with "timelines for reporting varying according to the seriousness and unexpectedness of the adverse drug reaction" (2004, p. 2624). Furthermore, Psaty et al. stated that "[a]lthough both manufacturers and the FDA can analyze the data and recommend actions such as label changes, additional warnings, or new studies, the FDA regulations largely focus on reporting procedures and, thus, leave unclear who is expected to initiate these actions" (p. 2624). Similarly to adverse reaction reports for Health Canada, the FDA's voluntary postmarking reporting system, MedWatch, is used to monitor the ongoing safety of marketed pharmaceuticals in the United States. The reports are triaged through the MedWatch program and then forwarded to the appropriate center (Pharmaceuticals, Biologics, Foods, or Veterinary). The work of reassessing pharmaceutical risks based on adverse drug reaction reports from hospitals, health care providers, and patients is accomplished primarily by the Division of Pharmacovigilance and Epidemiology, which employs data processing, epidemiology, and statistic staff in order to locate and evaluate patterns in reported adverse drug reactions. The division receives approximately 250,000 adverse reaction reports associated with pharmaceutical use annually. Approximately 25% of these reports are related to serious adverse reactions (Meadows, 2001).

3.4. FINANCIAL MATTERS AND REVIEWING PHARMACEUTICAL APPLICATIONS

In Canada as in the United States, the pharmaceutical industry itself funds the pharmaceutical-approval process through user fees. Beginning in the 1994–1995 fiscal year, there was a major shift in funding for the Therapeutic Products Directorate and the Biologics and Genetic Therapies Directorate, both branches of Health Canada that regulate pharmaceuticals (Lexchin, 2006b). "Cost recovery was to compensate for a reduction in direct government funding as the government sought to eliminate the budgetary deficit by cutting expenditures" (Lexchin, 2006b, p. 2216). Cost recovery was also seen as "a means of transferring some or all of the costs of a government activity from the general taxpayer to those who more directly benefit from or who 'trigger' that special activity" (KPMG Consulting LP, 2000, p. 2, as cited in Lexchin, 2006b, p. 2216). Under the new system, regulators were provided with greater access to resources in the form of funding to hire more staff, technology, and larger overall budgets with an implicit bargain that this would result in quicker turnaround times for pharmaceutical reviews. Since that time, pharmaceutical companies have paid fees for each new pharmaceutical that they submit for approval. In 2006 fees ranged from C$143,800 for a pharmaceutical for a single condition with a single dosage to C$212,000 for a pharmaceutical with two dosage forms (Lexchin, 2006b).

In the United States, the Prescription Drug User Fee Act of 1992 (PDUFA) was designed to help shorten the review time of both INDs and NDAs. The act allows the FDA to collect user fees from pharmaceutical companies as financial support used to fund the review process while also specifying that the FDA must review standard drug applications within 12 months of submission and priority applications within 6 months (Avorn, 2007). Applications for drugs similar to those on the market are considered standard, whereas priority applications represent drugs offering important advances in addition to existing treatments. Initially, the act allowed the FDA to levy user fees on pharmaceutical companies while also barring it from using those fees to monitor postmarketing safety. The PDUFA was reauthorized in 1997, but when Congress reauthorized it in 2002, about 5% of the fees were earmarked for postapproval safety monitoring (Hennessy and Strom, 2007). Avorn (2007) wrote that when the law was created in 1992, the FDA was regularly criticized for being too slow to approve new pharmaceuticals—especially new AIDS pharmaceuticals. In that climate, user fees seemed an ideal solution to eliminate perceived inefficiencies of the government and speed up the FDA "pipeline." The legislation, therefore, established strict time limits for pharmaceuticals to go through the FDA review process.

According to Guthrie (2007) and Avorn (2007), user fees from pharmaceutical companies account for over 40% of the FDA's annual budget, with projections of US$539 million in 2008. In Canada, user fees from pharmaceutical companies have accounted for 35 to 70% of the Therapeutic Products Directorate's annual budget of about C$70 million in the past 10 years (Kondro, 2002). As can be seen in figure 2, pharmaceutical user fees have comprised an increasing percentage of the total annual budgets of both the FDA's Center for Drug Evaluation and Research and the Therapeutic Products Directorate in Canada, beginning in 1992 and 1994, respectively.

As was just described, new prescription pharmaceuticals are expected to be developed and tested for quality, safety, and efficacy by the pharmaceutical industry in modern industrialized countries while little or no pharmaceutical testing is conducted by governmental organizations (Abraham, 2002a). Once completed, this data, most often funded by the manufacturers themselves, is often published in medical and scientific journals (Jacky Law, 2006). Such publications serve many purposes for the manufacturers, the most important of which are to function as evidence for approval of the pharmaceutical in question, to

FIGURE 2. Pharmaceutical user fees as percentage of total annual budgets of the Therapeutic Products Directorate in Canada, and the FDA's Center for Drug Evaluation and Research by year.

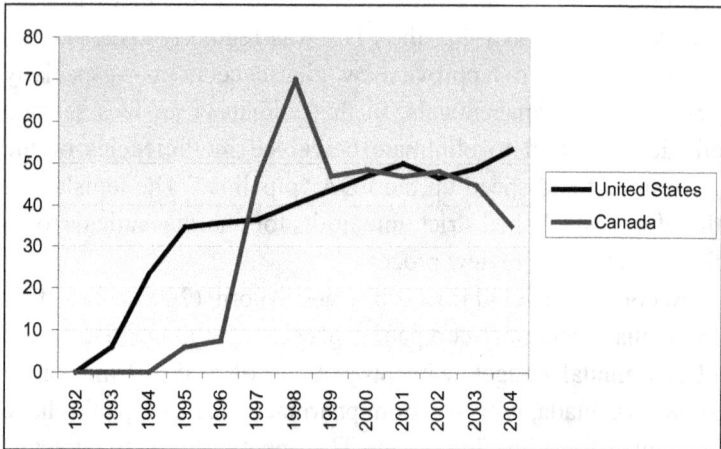

Source. Canadian data from Lexchin (2006b); U.S. data from Avorn (2007).

bolster excitement and support from potential physicians and patients, in the case that they require mobilization, to place pressure on approving authorities, and later on, to assist with sales.

Physicians have always been the direct link between pharmaceutical producers and patients, which is why the pharmaceutical industry spends billions of dollars on symposia and galas for physicians, offering incentives for prescriptions, and advertising and promoting their products to physicians (Conrad & Leiter, 2004). The role of physicians as "providers," however, is changing in the current medical marketplace, particularly due to direct-to-consumer advertising, which undermines the physicians' authority regarding which drugs to prescribe (Conrad & Leiter, 2004, p. 160). The Federal Drug Administration Modernization

Act of 1997 (United States) made drug advertising both more feasible and more attractive to pharmaceutical manufacturers. The changes in the Act, which allowed television and radio advertisements to name both the disorder and the drug's benefits without a lengthy summary of potential side effects and contraindications, are seen as the main reasons for annual spending on direct-to-consumer advertising for prescription pharmaceuticals increasing sixfold between 1996 and 2000 (Conrad & Leiter, 2004), contributing to maintenance of the pharmaceutical industry's ranking as the most profitable business in America (Lasser et al., 2002, p. 2219).[3]

Peter Lurie, deputy director of the Public Citizen's Health Research Group, wrote that "[i]n deciding whether pharmaceuticals are fit for prescribing to patients, the FDA states that it uses agency scientists to review the voluminous pharmaceutical submissions from sponsoring companies" (2006, p. 22). For about 30% of new pharmaceutical applications, the agency also assembles a meeting of an advisory committee comprised of nonagency experts whose opinions are expected to be impartial and in the interests of the public health (Lurie, 2006). As a result, many "outside" physicians and researchers participate in the FDA and Health Products and Food Branch approval councils by sitting on advisory committees, many of whom maintain direct and indirect links with the pharmaceutical companies and pharmaceuticals which they are expected to scrutinize objectively. As Abraham (2002b) noted, "[T]he pharmaceutical industry has been enthusiastic to foster direct or indirect financial links with expert advisors," some of whom have now "adopted the industry view that short regulatory review times are desirable because they deliver pharmaceuticals to patients in the fastest possible time" (p. 1499). In addition, the probability of regulators adapting and conforming to the interests and values of the industry is highly likely due to the fact that many regulatory officials receive their training from, and anticipate promotion back into, the industry after regulatory service via the so-called "revolving door" (Abraham, 2002b; Braithwaite, 1986).

3.5. LINKING INTERNATIONAL PHARMACEUTICAL CONTROL AGENCIES

Sales approval (as well as withdrawal) in the country of manufacture has importance not only for that particular country, but also for licensing decisions in other countries, although not always directly (Abraham & Lawton Smith, 2003). Because this book is concerned with similarities and differences between Canada and the United States regarding pharmaceutical regulation, it is imperative that any linkages, especially in the form of regulations or treaties, be analyzed as they relate to the two countries. In looking for and wanting to analyze these connections, however, what I found was that there is only one such set of loosely adhered-to regulations between Canada and the United States: the International Conference on Harmonization of Technical Requirements for Registration of Pharmaceuticals for Human Use (ICH). There appear to be no additional informal links between the HPFB and the FDA.

The ICH is a project which attempted to streamline pharmaceutical regulation internationally (Abraham & Lawton Smith, 2003). In the 1980s, what is today the European Union began harmonizing regulatory requirements for pharmaceutical approval. In 1989 Europe, Japan, and the United States began creating plans for harmonization, which resulted in ICH being officially created in April 1990 at a meeting in Brussels, Belgium (Abraham & Lawton Smith). In 1998 the secretariat of the ICH contended that "the urgent need" for harmonization was "impelled" by "the need to meet the public expectation that there should be a minimum of delay in making safe and efficacious treatments available to patients in need" (Idanpaan-Heikkila, 1998). As a result of the conference, the regulatory agencies of Central and Eastern Europe now automatically adopt ICH's scientific standards (Macinnes, 1997), and Canadian regulatory authorities have already adopted some (Health Canada, 1999). Meanwhile, supporters of ICH are lobbying the World Health Organization (WHO) to promote these standards throughout the developing world (Anonymous, 1992; Idanpaan-Heikkila, 1998). These standards will be discussed and examined further in chapter 5.

ENDNOTES

1. Of the 1,982 clinical trials conducted in Canada in 2005, 40 were inspected (Health Canada, 2006a).
2. Reporting requirements for lack of efficacy apply to "new drugs" as defined in Division 8 of the Food and Drugs Act.
3. The industry returned between 23 and 25% of its total revenue in profits in 2001–2002 (Pharmaceutical Research and Manufacturers of America [PhRMA] *Annual Report 2001–2002*, as cited in Goozner, 2004, p. 13).

CHAPTER 4

THE PHARMACEUTICAL
NETWORKS

4.1. APPROVING PEMOLINE FOR SALE

Some estimate that 4% to 12% of 6- to 12-year-olds in the
United States suffer from attention deficit hyperactivity disorder
(ADHD; Brown et al., 2001; Polanczyk, de Lima, Horta, Biederman, & Rohde, 2007). Similarly, in a review of general population studies of Canadian school-age children, the National
Longitudinal Survey of Children and Youth reported the best
prevalence estimates to range from 5 to 10% (Human Resources
Development Canada, 2002). As Willy, Manda, Shatin,
Drinkard, and Graham (2002) noted, many of these children will
be treated with some type of psychotropic medication. Pemoline (sold as Cylert by Abbott Laboratories) served as one such

pharmaceutical available for the treatment of ADHD after the drug's initial approval in Europe in the 1960s, in the United States in 1975, and in Canada in 1977. Clinical tests employing the pharmaceutical, a "central nervous system stimulant" for "undue fatigue" had been carried out since 1957 (Lienert & Janke, 1957; Lucas & Knowles, 1963; Meadley, 1965, p. 680) and supported financially by Abbott since 1967 (Talland & McGuire, 1967). Pemoline was not the first drug available for the treatment of ADHD, however, since Ritalin® was approved for ADHD treatment in 1955 in the United States (Mosholder, 2006).

In three large U.S. computerized databases covering youths under the age of 20, the treatment prevalence range[1] for pemoline rose approximately threefold from 0.08% to 0.19% in 1987 to 0.22% to 0.64% in 1996 (Safer & Zito, 2000). At the time of approval in the United States, delayed hypersensitivity[2] reactions involving the liver were noted to occur in 1% to 2% of patients receiving pemoline, leading to recommendations in the precautions section of the product monograph[3] to monitor liver enzyme levels periodically (Willy et al., 2002). In the first year of U.S. marketing, one case of serious pemoline-related hepatotoxicity was reported to the FDA (Willy et al.). Subsequently, reports of serious cases of pemoline-related hepatotoxicity appeared in the literature, including cases of acute liver failure (Adcock, MacElroy, Wolford, & Farrington, 1998; Berkovitch, Pope, Phillips, & Koren, 1995; Elitsur, 1990; Hochman, Woodard, & Cohen, 1998; Jaffe, 1989; Marotta & Roberts, 1998; McCurry & Cronquist, 1997; Nehra, Mullick, Ishak, & Zimmerman, 1990; Page, Bernstein, Janicki, & Michelli, 1974; Patterson, 1984; Pratt & Dubois, 1990; Rosh, Dellert, Narkewich, Birnbarum, & Whittington, 1998; Safer, Zito, & Gardner, 2001; Sterling, Kane, & Grace, 1996, as cited in Willy et al., 2002). There was no change in the prescribing

recommendations for the drug from the time of approval, however, illustrating the creation and stability of the black box which
had been formed around it and which made pemoline a stable,
accepted treatment for ADHD. The FDA and Health Canada
were aware of adverse reaction reports, but no specific action was
taken by the governing bodies until 1996. In Canada, 17 adverse
reaction reports had been sent to the HPFB beginning in 1988,
while in the United States, the number remains unknown.

4.2. WITHDRAWING PEMOLINE FROM THE MARKET

The accumulation of reports of liver harm and failure caused
by pemoline finally prompted a pharmaceutical-company labeling change in December of 1996, about 20 years after its initial
approval, which was accompanied by a "Dear Health Care Provider" letter to U.S. physicians. The risk of liver failure with
pemoline use was highlighted in a black box warning—the
strongest warning that the FDA requires—on its product monograph, and the pharmaceutical was shifted from first-line to
second-line therapy for ADHD by the FDA. New recommendations were added specifying baseline and biweekly liver enzyme
monitoring (Pizzuti, 1996). A similar labeling change was sent to
Canadian physicians in 1997, warning of potential liver failure,
following reports of 11 related deaths in the United States (since
1975) and a number of cases in other foreign countries. The letter sent to physicians by Health Canada also included a warning that Cylert not be considered as a first-line pharmaceutical
therapy for ADHD alongside Ritalin (Keung and Daly, 1998).
By September of the same year, the Medicines Control Agency
of the United Kingdom withdrew the government license for
pemoline distribution in the United Kingdom due to "serious
hepatotoxicity" (Medicines Control Agency, 1997).

By December of 1998, pemoline was acknowledged as being under review by Health Canada's HPFB after being linked to liver failure in 13 patients in Canada and the United States since initial approval, signaling the slow breakdown of the previously "assumed to be solid" black box (Immen, 1998). "We're doing a risk assessment on it right now to see how best to manage the risk, but the pharmaceutical will stay on the market with warning information," said Dr. Brian Gillespie, senior medical adviser to Health Canada's bureau of pharmaceutical assessments (Immen, 1998, p. A13). By September of 1999, Health Canada followed the lead of the United Kingdom and withdrew pemoline from the Canadian market due to its review concerning hepatotoxicity (Health Canada Advisory, 1999). The conclusion was based on a number of considerations, including the fact that

> despite explicit warnings in the product monograph and labelling information regarding the risk of severe liver damage, worldwide case reports of liver failure necessitating transplantation or resulting in death continued; there was no evidence that liver damage caused by the pharmaceutical was predictable or reversible; that other, safer treatment alternatives were available; and that a satisfactory response to the Therapeutic Products Program's request for specific evidence to support the safety of the pharmaceutical's continued use was not provided by the manufacturer. (Hogan, 2000, p. 3)

There was no direct mention however, of the existence of other pharmaceuticals for ADHD treatment which could be given once a day. According to Public Citizen's Health Research Group, "[T]he main initial appeal of pemoline to clinicians was that it allowed once-a-day dosing, as opposed to multiple daily doses which might raise logistical problems especially for children in school during the day" (2005). However, due to the development of once-a-day dosing of other standard stimulant medications, this was no longer a unique characteristic, but rather one which was shared by other medications (assumed to be less harmful) such as Ritalin-SR®, Adderall XR®, Dexedrine®, and Concerta®. In the United States by contrast, in June of 1999, a second "Dear Health Care Provider" letter was mailed by the manufacturer to physicians concerning pemoline hepatotoxicity indicating that there were additional major adverse drug reactions resulting from the pharmaceutical and recommending increased restrictions to its use (Pizzuti, 1999). Presumably because of the manufacturer's warning letters, the sales of pemoline in the United States declined markedly between 1996 and 1999, although in 1999, its sales still represented approximately 2% to 3% of the total U.S. sales of methylphenidate, amphetamine, and pemoline—the top ADHD pharmaceuticals (Greenhill, 2000, as cited in Safer et al., 2001). Still, in 1999, Copley Pharmaceutical Inc. applied for, and received, FDA approval to manufacture generic pemoline, a therapeutically equivalent compound to Abbott Laboratories' Cylert. And in September of 2000, the FDA once again approved another manufacturer's—Watson Pharmaceuticals Inc.—application to manufacture generic pemoline tablets.

In March of 2005, Public Citizen petitioned the FDA to immediately ban Cylert and all generic versions of pemoline due to evidence that the drug caused liver failure and that it had no unique advantage over other drugs used to treat the same condition. At the time, physicians in the United States were still prescribing about 117,000 doses of Cylert and its generic equivalents per year, the petition said. At least 13 patients had died since 1975 while on the pharmaceutical, and reports given to the FDA showed that at least 193 patients have suffered serious consequences from the pharmaceutical, noted Dr. Peter Lurie, deputy director of the organization (Public Citizen's Health

Research Group, 2005). The petition noted that while the United Kingdom and Canada removed the pharmaceutical from the market, the FDA, stating that the pharmaceutical still offered favorable treatment for some, instead chose twice to stiffen warnings on the pharmaceutical's label (Public Citizen's Health Research Group, 2005). Notably, Public Citizen's petition to the FDA angered the Narcolepsy Network and its many members who claimed to have benefitted greatly from the medication. The pharmaceutical had been employed off-label (outside the scope of the approved uses of the pharmaceutical) by an estimated 10,000 Americans diagnosed with the sleep disorders of narcolepsy and idiopathic hypersomnia. In an untreated state, both disorders are characterized by excessive sleepiness and sleep attacks during the day.

Shortly after the Public Citizen petition was filed, Abbott Laboratories announced that it would discontinue marketing and sales of Cylert for economic reasons: "The pharmaceutical's sales this year will be less than $1 million," company representatives noted (Knowles, 2005, p. 62). There was no response from the six companies selling generic versions of the drug. By October of 2005, the FDA was not recalling the pharmaceutical, but was instead allowing pharmacies to sell their remaining stock as doctors still using it switched patients to other treatments. At this time, the FDA noted that all companies producing generic pemoline had also agreed to stop sales and marketing and that "Cylert would remain available until current supplies ran out," angering consumer advocates who had been arguing the pharmaceutical was too dangerous to be sold (Knowles, 2005, p. 62). In a subsequent *Alert for Healthcare Professionals*, the agency wrote that

> given the availability of multiple other pharmaceutical treatments for ADHD, including one that is not scheduled

[restricted] and several products that can be given once a day, the FDA has concluded that the risk of liver failure with this pharmaceutical outweighs the potential benefits. (Food and Drug Administration, 2005b)

4.3. APPROVING TOLCAPONE FOR SALE

Parkinson's disease is an age-related progressive neurodegenerative disorder estimated to affect about 1% of adults aged 60 years and older (Keating & Lyseng-Williamson, 2005; Leegwater-Kim & Waters, 2006). The pharmaceutical compound levodopa increases dopamine, a hormone and neurotransmitter in the brain, and is the mainstay therapy for patients with the disease, which involves a decrease in dopamine levels in the brain (Borges, 2003). Within 5 years of starting levodopa therapy, however, about 50% of patients will experience motor function fluctuations, or "wearing off" effects in response to treatment, making levodopa treatment decreasingly effective with time (Keating & Lyseng-Williamson, 2005). Research has shown that this is due to a molecule in the blood called catechol-*o*-methyltransferase enzyme (COMT), which is known to break down levodopa (Keating & Lyseng-Williamson, 2005).

Tolcapone (Tasmar) was the first drug known to selectively break down COMT, extending the lifespan of levodopa, and as a result, is prescribed to Parkinson's patients alongside levodopa treatment. In fact, studies consistently found that significant improvements in "on" and "off" times,[4] ranging from 0.9 to 1.8 hours, were observed with tolcapone, with results varying slightly between studies and dosages (Baas et al., 1997; Kieburtz & Hubble, 2000, S42; Rajput, Martin, Saint-Hilaire, Dorflinger, & Peder, 1997). As an inhibitor, tolcapone helps to provide more consistent and effective relief for the symptoms of Parkinson's disease, which includes uncontrollable tremors, stiffness, poor balance, and a shuffling walk during "off times" but that disappear during "on" times (Leegwater-Kim & Waters, 2006). It was developed in the laboratories of Hoffman-La Roche Inc. in the early 1980s (Borroni, Borgulya, & Zurcher, 1998; Da Prada, Keller, Pieri, Kettler, & Haefely, 1984) and launched in Canada and the European Union in late 1997 and in the United States in early 1998 (Keating & Lyseng-Williamson, 2005). A second COMT inhibitor, entacapone, was approved in 1999 in the United States and Canada in 2001 (Food and Drug Administration, 1999a; Health Canada, 2008).

In clinical trials of tolcapone, liver chemistry tests were elevated more than three times above the upper limit of normal in approximately 1% of patients administered the 100mg dose and in approximately 3% of patients administered the 200mg dose. These observations led to the recommendation that periodic monitoring of patients' liver function be performed by physicians (Borges, 2005). Coupled with significant numbers of patient dropouts due to adverse reactions in premarketing clinical trials[5] and other serious adverse reactions, such as adverse effects on cardiac function and diarrhea (itself a symptom of hepatic damage[6]), the pharmaceutical barely passed the FDA approval process, which was conditional upon 18 amendments and numerous postapproval studies expected to be completed by the manufacturer. It is not known whether these requirements were completed since most of them stated that "the sponsor should..." not that the sponsor was "required to" (Center for Drug Evaluation and Research, Medical Reviews, 1998, p. 10). Interestingly, only 647 patients had been exposed to the pharmaceutical for at least a year prior to its approval (Division of Neuropharmacological Drug Products—Food and Drug Administration, 1997). These factors led to the creation of a weak and shaky black box of tolcapone, wherein its approval did not lead to the pharmaceutical being unanimously prescribed and lauded as a breakthrough drug.

4.4. WITHDRAWING TOLCAPONE OFF THE CANADIAN MARKET

Postmarketing surveillance studies conducted by a team of neurologists and gastroenterologists in Switzerland noted three instances, including one in Canada, of acute liver failure resulting in death stemming from tolcapone use beginning in September of 1998 (Assal, Spahr, Hadengue, Rubbici-Brandt, & Burkhard, 1998), and eight cases of serious liver injury after 100,000 patients had been prescribed tolcapone worldwide (Health Canada Advisory, 1998). For this reason, the pharmaceutical was withdrawn from the market in Canada and the European Union in late 1998 (Borroni, Cesura, Gatti, & Gasser, 2001), and a black box warning was issued in the United States (Hoffman-LaRoche Laboratories, 1998). Due to tolcapone's known interference with liver enzymes, the warning advised prescribing physicians to perform routine liver enzyme monitoring on patients. As Watkins (2000, S51) wrote,

> [B]ecause a patient who experiences a [liver enzyme] type of liver injury typically becomes jaundiced early in the course of the illness, this type of problem is usually recognized in time to stop the medication and avoid serious liver dysfunction.

Interestingly, none of the patients with severe reactions to the pharmaceutical had been regularly monitored as suggested. In contrast, no case of severe liver dysfunction has been reported in patients who were monitored according to labeling recommendations (Watkins, 2000).

By April of 2004, suspension of the tolcapone marketing authorization in the European Union had been lifted on the recommendation of the Committee on Proprietary Medicinal Products 6 years after its withdrawal (Konopka & Czlonkowski, 2005). Having received additional clinical safety data from the manufacturer, as well as "having better insight and understanding of safety concerns relating to hepatitis and neuroleptic malignant-like syndrome," the committee recommended the lifting of the suspension provided that the following three conditions were followed: more stringent liver function monitoring, contraindication in patients with certain conditions, as well as restricting prescribing ability to "physicians experienced in the management of advanced Parkinson's disease" (European Medicines Agency, 2004).

Since tolcapone's submission to strict FDA regulations, no further cases of liver failure have been reported, as the regulations have seriously limited the use of tolcapone in patients (Borges, 2003). Nonetheless, by February of 2006, the FDA had approved further safety labeling revisions for tolcapone in order to warn of the risk of severe hepatocellular injury, including liver failure leading to death, associated with its use (Waknine, 2006). This further adds to the illustration of the tolcapone black box as unsteady and partial to failure in the United States, much as it was in Canada.

ENDNOTES

1. The treatment prevalence range is comprised of American youths under the age of 20 who were on pemoline therapy as a percentage of all American youths under the age of 20 in both 1987 and 1996.

2. Delayed hypersensitivity reactions are undesirable (often inflammatory) reactions produced by the healthy immune system 2 to 3 days after treatment with a compound new to the system.

3. A product monograph is a scientific document about the pharmaceutical compound that describes the properties, claims, indications, and conditions of use for the pharmaceutical and that contains any other information that may be required for its optimal, safe, and effective use. The product monograph never contains promotional materials (Health Canada, 2007).

4. When patients take Parkinson's disease medications, they usually notice that their symptoms cease for hours at a time (termed "on times"), then return (termed "off times"). Symptoms also return during the wearing off period, when Parkinson's treatments become less effective. Moving back and forth between "on" and "off" times is a reality for Parkinson's disease patients. "On" times can also be accompanied by side effects called dyskinesias, wherein the patient experiences sudden jerky or uncontrolled movements of the limbs and neck (Tasmar Product Monograph, 2006).

5. Trial withdrawal rates ranged from 18% (200mg per day) to 20% (100mg per day) for patients taking tolcapone (Center for Drug Evaluation and Research, Medical Reviews, 1998, p. 46).

6. From Castillo et al., 2001.

CHAPTER 5

ANALYSIS

Studying up does not mean being submitted to the agenda of those we study: what some disgruntled scientists conclude from our research remains their business, not ours. As far as I can tell...they might have concluded that the white purity of science should never be sullied by the dark and greasy fingers of mere sociologists.

—Latour (2005, p. 100)

In his pioneering book, the founder of the sociology of science, Ludwig Fleck, provided an excellent description of the genesis of scientific fact:

> To give an accurate historical account of a scientific discipline is impossible. It is as if we wanted to record in writing the natural course of an excited conversation among several persons all speaking simultaneously among themselves and each clamouring to make himself

heard, yet which nevertheless permitted a consensus to crystallize. (Fleck, 1981, p. 15)

Although it is imperative to acknowledge the divide between one reality and its many interpretations as actor network theory (ANT) does in its discussion of multiplicities, one must nonetheless assemble one collective story comprised of each actor's history and viewpoints for the purpose of combined analysis in a written work such as a book. For obvious reasons, I could not write and analyze a separate history of each pharmaceutical from the perspective of each actor involved in each network. Rather, what I had to do was examine every actor and allow them to "speak," yet assemble all of these discourses into one collective analysis. This chapter serves as this collectivity in its analysis of each pharmaceutical's history in Canada and the United States based on each actor's historical experience from preapproval to withdrawal. After all, "the most productive way to create new narratives has been to follow the development of an innovation" (Latour, 1993, as cited in John Law, 1999, p. 111).

My employment of ANT strongly influenced how I researched, assembled, and decided to present each story and the actors involved in it. After all, the theoretical and methodological framework provided by ANT focuses on networks, their connections, and the work that happens between actors. It is with mapping these associations and the worknet that emerges between them that I discovered new, important actors, such as adverse reaction reports, and how they became part of the story. The sort of action that was flowing from one actor to the other was most often in the form of documents which relayed information and evidence, monetary exchanges, or, in the case of the pharmaceuticals themselves, the risks and benefits conferred by their associated treatments.

A crucial aspect of ANT is a sense of skepticism and questioning of the status quo. In effect, this manifests itself as the "unpacking" of black boxes, which appear as taken-for-granted facts and technologies comprising nodes in networks. Where possible, I attempted to research, examine, and in short, uncover as much information as possible about each node and what factors influenced and added to the functioning or disintegration of its network. For example, when Health Canada actively withdrew tolcapone off of the market after a relatively small number of patient deaths compared to those caused by other medications, I researched and examined each of the actors involved in the network and what had changed to cause the instability and eventual failure of the tolcapone network. In this analysis, I examine each pharmaceutical and changes in its functioning, the manufacturer's actions, the scientific literature and its prevailing treatment of the pharmaceutical, adverse reaction reports, the medical profession, and, lastly, the patients and their impact on the decision to withdraw and the impact of said decision on the patients. It is by following the work and actions leading from one node to another that the network begins to take shape and through which one begins to uncover and understand the atmosphere and the actors comprising that network. When both the Canadian and American networks are sketched out, one can slowly begin to understand why the pharmaceutical was treated so differently in each one. After all, an understanding of the prevailing climate in each country helps to better elucidate why decisions to withdraw were or were not made by regulatory authorities.

5.1. DISCUSSING THE NETWORKED ACTORS

Western medicine is commonly seen as a cohesive discipline in which views, beliefs, and forms of reasoning are shared, particularly in contrast with non-Western conventional medical practice. In their work entitled *Differences in Medicine*, Berg and Mol (1998) expose this illusion with a multidisciplinary and multicultural anthology of essays which reveals the considerable variation in which practitioners of "conventional" Western medicine manage bodies, results, statistics, and conversations with patients. As a result, what had been seen as a single and uniform field of practice gradually becomes an assembly of highly divergent practices (Berg & Mol, 1998). The cases of pemoline and tolcapone may also initially appear to exist as cohesive compounds treated and employed in uniform ways internationally. Although it can be said that each compound consists of the same chemical formula and the same dosing instructions resulting in a uniform field of practice, the way in which it is actually seen, treated, and worked with varies widely. This assembly of highly divergent practices results from the creation of what has been termed the *pharmaceutical pipeline*, whose purpose is to transform new biological compounds into new medicines through a series of stages, including laboratory and clinical research, the application and satisfaction of government policy and regulatory approval, patent procurement, and marketing (Mather, 2005, p. 1324; Mather, 2006). The metaphor of the pharmaceutical pipeline situates the behaviors and practices of actors in the approval and marketing sectors involved in bringing each new pharmaceutical to the medicine cabinet. Considering that it takes about 13 years for a pharmaceutical to progress through the course, it, too, acquires indeterminate identities and statuses during its development time (Mather, 2006).

Mather's (2006) examination of a compound's sequence of temporal stages and phases as it progresses through the pipeline is of immense value regarding the subject in question: Each pharmaceutical begins in research laboratories as a "biological material with interesting properties" and goes on to either become a new compound ready to be altered in order to comprise other compounds or one ready for testing on animals (p. 86). After passing the requirements of further laboratory testing, the candidate compound then enters the medical clinic where it is subjected to further testing, this time on humans, in order to determine that it is safe and effective for its intended use. At the completion of the clinical testing stage, the pharmaceutical then "enters the regulatory arena as a candidate medicine. Given regulatory approval, the pharmaceutical entity becomes a certified pharmaceutical" (Mather, 2006, p. 86). The dissection of each pharmaceutical's route through the pipeline encompasses time, an assortment of various other actors, as well as a multiplicity of physical settings such as wet labs, dry labs, clinics, boardrooms, financial markets, and government offices. It is with mapping these nodes, their associations, and the network that emerges between them that this book is concerned. The concept of networks or worknets focuses on the work done at each node and its connection with the next in order to move the pharmaceutical from one point in the pharmaceutical pipeline to the subsequent one. After all, researchers at the laboratory and in the clinic must do work and produce results which are passed on along with the compound to those comprising the next phase of the pipeline at the approval stage.

Although Mather did not explicitly identify as a practitioner of ANT, I believe that his perspective is similar to, and harmonious with, that of ANT for multiple reasons, including the fact that he believed that pharmaceuticals themselves do things and possess "indeterminate identities" as they pass through the pipeline (Mather, 2006, p. 85). These indeterminate identities arise because "the labels for and properties of a prospective medicine change depending upon when and where it is in the drug pipeline" resulting in a certain identity and "definitive status" in each setting of each stage (Mather, pp. 85–86). This viewpoint can be seen as largely synonymous with ANT's concept of "multiplicities" in actors' identities, although this word was not used specifically by Mather. Mather also wrote about physical settings in the pharmaceutical pipeline as being associated with "social worlds," which are "inhabited by actors who share regular mutual responses to the context of their lives and who form some kind of organization or network" (Mather, p. 86). Although this view tends to focus more on physical settings than actual actors in a network or their resulting nodes, it nonetheless is described very similarly to what ANT scholars term *the actor network*. Lastly, what is referred to by ANT scholars as "translation" or more colloquially as the "glue" keeping actors within a network, appears very similar to what Mather called "boundary objects" wherein "concepts, ideas, or objects that bridge the interests, actions, and understandings of actors from different domains" serve as the links "allying interests and understandings" and in short, keep networks together (p. 87).

The similarities in both theoretical frameworks allow their employment concurrently in analyzing the networks of pemoline and tolcapone. The pipeline metaphor is useful in this study because it conveys imagery of the existence and relative locations of many of the actors who emerged from my research into both pharmaceuticals' histories. Through this, the pipeline serves to locate both pemoline and tolcapone in the larger worlds of all pharmaceuticals being discovered, tested, approved, and withdrawn. The pipeline metaphor also allows one to situate the many stages and actors within them, which serve to work on and influence the pharmaceuticals as they travel through. These static actors "see" the pharmaceutical in different ways depending on the actors' location and job in the pipeline, which in turn elucidates the multiplicities of identities conferred on the pharmaceuticals themselves.

Congruent with Mather's approach, ANT sees pharmaceutical entities in the pipeline as not simply transforming themselves, but rather relying on actors[1] in physical settings to perform routines that serve to alter and regulate the pharmaceuticals both physically and conceptually. Mather (2006) wrote that

> the drug entities in the pipeline do not transform themselves; actors in physical settings perform routines that serve to alter the pharmaceutical entities both physically and conceptually. Actors from the domain of science work in wet and dry labs while actors from the domains of medicine and industry perform in clinics and boardrooms, respectively. (p. 86)

Where the two theoretical frameworks diverge however, is that ANT sees pharmaceuticals as possessing agency and, in turn, causing the actors around them to do things in response to the pharmaceuticals themselves who change over time. Mather's framework, in contrast, leans towards a more human-centered approach to agency wherein "movement across the stages of the pipe creates a social biography, a series of transformations made possible and actualized by human agency" (2005, p. 1324). Mather acknowledged, however, that "a drug has social agency because it can influence, alter and reinforce patterns of personal behaviour, and social relations and interaction" (2006, p. 86).

Actors do not always act on their own agency. According to the ANT viewpoint, it was not solely pemoline or tolcapone which simply transformed themselves from "nonapprovable" to "approvable" compounds, but rather it was scientists, statisticians, and trial designers who did their work by responding to the compounds in order for those in governmental organizations to be able to do their work by examining the resulting scripts and evidence. Furthermore, other important nonhuman actors were strongly involved in the processes of approval and withdrawal and those in between—they will also be analyzed in this chapter. These include scientific publications, user fees, marketing practices, adverse reaction reports, and Canadian and American regulation policies. Although Mather did not specifically examine the actions and influence of nonhuman actors directly on the pharmaceuticals travelling through pharmaceutical pipelines, they will be analyzed in this book in order to further elucidate each actor's role on each pharmaceutical's travels through the pipeline. After all, a basic tenant of ANT is that both human and nonhuman actors be analyzed symmetrically because they all influence other actors in their networks equally.

The image of a pipeline may appear to suggest that all pharmaceutical compounds proceed through a standardized process. Although each pharmaceutical may be seen as going through a pipeline, the histories of the pharmaceuticals in question demonstrate that each pharmaceutical's pipeline is not identical, but rather unique, resulting in many divergent pipelines for many pharmaceuticals. In addition, it is important to note that the pipeline is by no means solely conducive to one-way flow. Rather, the pharmaceutical development and approval process may require multiple trips upstream and downstream in order to secure whatever information or authorization is required further upstream, as was the case for both pemoline and tolcapone prior to receiving approval. According to both Canadian and American reviewers' documents, multiple amendments were required in each case, with the pharmaceutical being returned "downstream" to the manufacturer for further testing and analysis prior to being resent "upstream" for consideration for approval once more.

5.2. THE ROLE OF SCIENTIFIC PUBLICATIONS

A crucial set of actors involved in the approval and withdrawal of arguably all pharmaceuticals today is that of medical and scientific publications. This critical role of scientific publications and how they factor into the realm of pharmaceutical governance and marketing in today's medical culture is influenced strongly by sources of funding for scientific research. As was mentioned in chapter 3, what is employed in investigating and scrutinizing a pharmaceutical for potential approval is not solely its manufacturer's data, but also a limited number of scientific publications most often funded by the manufacturer themselves. Considering that pharmaceutical makers have vested interests, economical or otherwise, in the approval and sales of pharmaceuticals, any data provided or funded by them may be inherently biased. Furthermore, Freeman (1976) offered a jolting passage on the decision-making practices of journal editors scrutinizing manuscripts:

> Scepticism is warranted in reading the results of *any* study. We should remember that the editors of a journal do not review the raw data. They decide to print a submitted manuscript based upon the author's reputation, the relevance and organization of the material, and the opinions of referees (who don't see the raw data either). Editors *assume* that the investigator actually did what he described. Unfortunately, this is not always true and may produce an undetermined amount of bias. Positive results are also more likely to be submitted for publication than are negative ones. (p. 20, italics in original)

For various individual reasons, all of the actors introduced previously in the examination of pemoline and tolcapone worked together to produce and make possible the approval and sale of both pharmaceuticals, wherein each individual pharmaceutical is a multiplicity of those with vested interests in it. It is reasonable to argue then, as did McKinlay in 1981 in his milestone article outlining "the seven stages in the career of a medical innovation," that the success of an innovation is not based upon its intrinsic worth, whether it is measurably effective, as determined by experimentation, but rather upon the power of the multiple interests that sponsor and maintain it, despite the absence or inadequacy of objective empirical support for it. The power of such interests "is also evident in their ability to impede the development of alternative practices (for which there may also be considerable observational support) that could conceivably threaten an activity in which there is already considerable investment" such as self-reporting any adverse events by the manufacturers themselves or attempting to surpass competitors' sales (McKinlay, 1981, p. 398).

The attempt to impede the development of alternative practices is evident with Abbott Laboratories' funding of a study comparing the efficacy and safety of methylphenidate (Ritalin) and pemoline in the treatment of children with attention deficit hyperactivity disorder (ADHD) in 2000 (Andriola, 2000). The study noted that

> in 1998 Ritalin constituted 70% of the market...in order to compare the efficacy of these drugs in a large population of children and to assess adverse events associated with their administration, we conducted a retrospective descriptive study of 500 children treated for ADHD.

Not surprisingly, the results found that "a higher percentage of pemoline than Ritalin-treated children had an excellent clinical response" (Andriola, 2000, p. 208). By the year 2000, pemoline had been withdrawn from the United Kingdom and Canada, but was still available in the United States, so both the timing and content of the study suggest that it was published as a desperate attempt to increase sales of the pharmaceutical. In a similar effort to increase the number of patients being treated with pemoline, the manufacturer funded another study in 1999 designed to determine whether adults with ADHD benefited from pemoline use, which up until that point had been largely concentrated on children's treatment (Wilens et al., 1999). The results of the study stated that "treatment with pemoline was effective in the amelioration of ADHD symptoms" and that "the results support the continuity of pharmacologic responsivity of this syndrome across the lifespan" (Wilens et al., 1999, p. 261). Both studies exemplify action and funding taken on by the manufacturer in order to increase sales of pemoline at the expense of other pharmaceuticals developed for the same condition, in effect impeding the use and development of alternative practices.

A similar situation was observed with the drug tolcapone. In the 1990s, Orion, a Finnish pharmaceutical company, and Hoffmann-La Roche, its Swiss counterpart, were both simultaneously developing very similar anti-Parkinson's disease pharmaceuticals: Both were catechol-o-methyltransferase enzyme (COMT) inhibitors aimed at relieving patients with Parkinson's disease of levodopa-induced side effects. Coupled with similar efficacy and price, the pharmaceuticals were considered strong competitors. In 2001 Orion funded a comparative toxicological study on the hepatic safety of entacapone (Orion's pharmaceutical) and tolcapone (Hoffmann-La Roche's Tasmar). Not surprisingly, the study's authors concluded that "the toxicological profile of the two COMT inhibitors, entacapone and tolcapone, differed from each other, tolcapone—unlike entacapone— showed hepatotoxicity" (Haasio, Sopanen, Vaalavirta, Linden, & Heinonen, 2001, p. 79). Another interesting study was funded by both manufacturers in 2001 in order to compare the long-term tolerability and efficacy of both tolcapone and entacapone in patients with Parkinson's disease. The study's findings included the following: "[T]olcapone appears to have greater and longer efficacy with regard to motor symptoms, 'off' time, and change in levodopa requirements than entacapone. These findings indicate that tolcapone continues to have a place in the treatment of advanced Parkinson's disease." The authors continued, however, by stating that "the risks associated with this drug, particularly hepatic injury, and the requirement for rigorous blood monitoring, need to be considered when choosing an appropriate treatment for patients with advanced Parkinson's disease" (Factor, Molho, Feustel, Brown, & Evans, 2001, p. 295). Since both manufacturers funded the study, it is likely that the resulting article, rather than serve to impede the sales of either pharmaceutical, was published in order to focus on the benefits of each in a likely effort to provide scientific support for both entacapone and tolcapone's respective benefits—tolcapone worked better but also had greater adverse effects, a finding echoed in other publications (Kieburtz & Hubble, 2000). It appears that both manufacturers chose to coexist rather than be outdone by the other, especially in existing markets where both are still approved for sale and perhaps more suitable for different patient subsets.

In any discussion on scientific literature, it is important to consider the plethora of studies demonstrating that manufacturer-sponsored research has a far greater likelihood of yielding positive results compared to non-manufacturer-funded research (Cho & Bero, 1996; Davidson, 1986; Jacky Law, 2006; Stelfox, Chua, O'Rourke, & Detsky, 1998) as well as studies demonstrating that increased corporate involvement leads to increased secrecy in medical research (Blumenthal, Campbell, Causino, &

Seashore, 1996; Blumenthal, Causino, Campbell, & Seashore, 1996; Rosenberg, 1996). Support for this statement is found in a disturbing study in *The New England Journal of Medicine*, which revealed that 96% of medical experts who published studies or other articles supporting the use of certain controversial blood-pressure pharmaceuticals had financial ties with companies that make them, while only 37% of those who wrote articles critical of the pharmaceuticals had such ties (Stelfox et al., 1998). Considering the fact that publications serve as valuable sources of evidence for pharmaceutical reviewers considering approval or withdrawal of compounds, such influence into the published outcomes of research findings is highly controversial. After all, the general tone of the author towards the pharmaceutical, whether supportive or critical, could influence very important regulatory decisions.

In order to determine the overall tone of journal articles on both pemoline and tolcapone prior to approval and onwards, a database was constructed for each pharmaceutical. The constructed database contained all journal articles for all therapeutic uses of each of the pharmaceuticals from relevant time periods. Each article in each database was analyzed regarding and categorized according to its overall tone—whether supportive, critical, or neutral—towards the pharmaceutical in question. The results are displayed in figures 3 and 4.

As is evidenced by both figures 3 and 4, at the time of approval, as well as during the preceding years, journal articles on both pharmaceuticals had a tendency to be overwhelmingly supportive in tone towards the pharmaceuticals in question. When submitted as evidence for pharmaceutical approval, this would undoubtedly serve to positively influence reviewers' impressions towards the pharmaceuticals. Regarding withdrawal, figure 3 illustrates the substantial increase in critical

FIGURE 3. The number of journal articles in the pemoline database categorized by overall tone of article, by year.

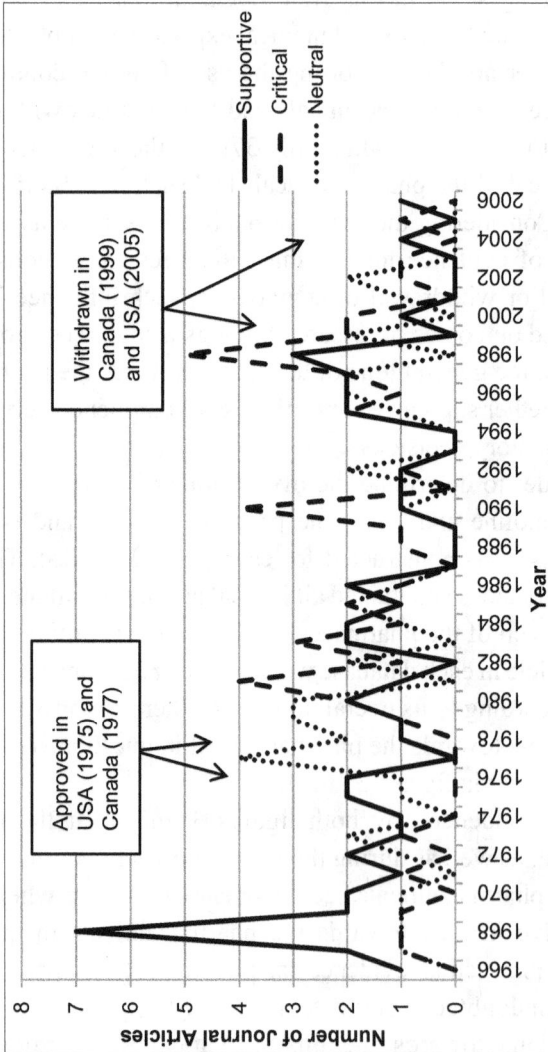

FIGURE 4. The number of journal articles in the tolcapone database categorized by overall tone of article, by year.

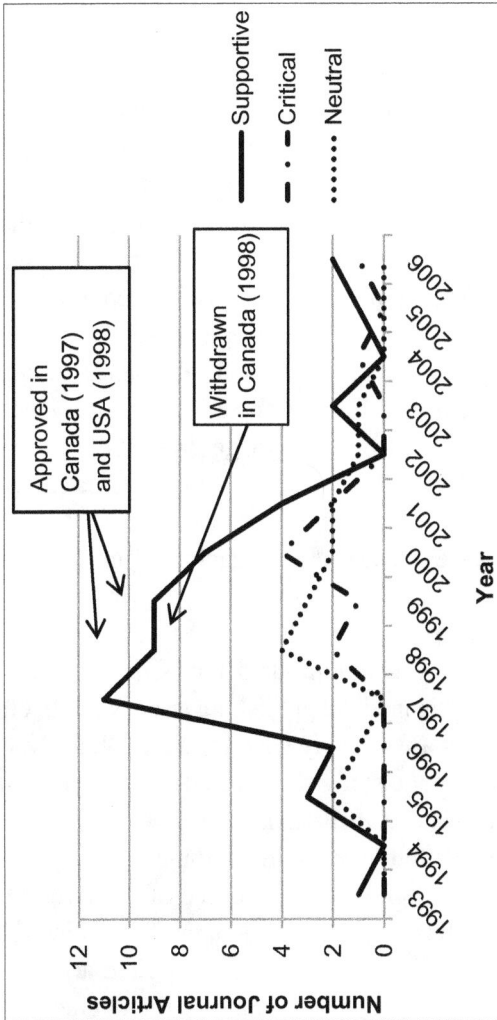

articles and decrease in supportive articles on pemoline shortly before and during withdrawal times of the pharmaceutical by both countries. Figure 4, however, displays a phenomenon of interest. Even though tolcapone was withdrawn from Canada just one year after approval, which was the same year that the Food and Drug Administration (FDA) was in the process of approving it, journal articles on tolcapone were overwhelmingly supportive towards the pharmaceutical.

Due to evidence from other studies suggesting that authors' sources of funding may impact their results, I decided to further examine the most influential, or heavily cited, articles published on pemoline and tolcapone. In order to do this, I performed a cited-reference search of the Web of Science. A search of all articles published in the Web of Science with *pemoline* in the title—and not limited by language or article type—resulted in 288 articles. Using these articles, a cross-tabulation was created to indicate the 10 most cited articles. These articles were then examined for evidence of manufacturers' involvement or support in the research. Unfortunately, this information was not always available, particularly with the older publications. This is by no means a unique finding but is rather a reflection of a larger problem in medical publishing as a whole. In effect, affiliations, such as a university's name, were often given as solely locations where the study was carried out, while no financial or employment-related affiliations were given.

With regards to the pemoline findings, although seven of the articles did not acknowledge a source of support, the three that did had direct links to the manufacturer of pemoline: Abbott Laboratories. These included the 3rd most cited article which was cited a total of 107 times in the index, the 6th most cited article which was cited 72 times, and the 10th most cited article which was cited 46 times. The authors of the 3rd and 6th most cited articles were stated as employed by Abbott Laboratories, while the 10th most cited article's author acknowledged the manufacturer for supporting the research leading to the publication. A search of all articles published in the Web of Science with *tolcapone* in the title—and not limited by language or article type—resulted in 166 articles. Using these articles, a second cross-tabulation was created to indicate the 10 most cited articles in this subset. These articles were then also examined for evidence of manufacturers' involvement or support in the research. Nine of the 10 articles had direct links to the manufacturer Hoffmann-La Roche, and not surprisingly, all were supportive of tolcapone. Only the 6th most cited article, cited 74 times, was not linked to the manufacturer and it was not supportive of tolcapone. Rather it was among the first articles to warn of a possible link between tolcapone use and acute liver failure (Assal et al., 1998). Of the nine supportive articles cited a combined total of 755 times, six articles acknowledged support from Hoffmann-La Roche, while three more stated that all authors were employed by the manufacturer. Of note is the most highly cited article, cited 136 times, which acknowledged that the "study was designed and funded by Hoffmann-La Roche" and was authored by the "Tolcapone Fluctuator Study Group I" comprised of 33 investigators throughout the United States (Kurth et al., 1997). Considering the timing of the publication, it was likely employed by the manufacturer as evidence to support its application for approval in both Canada and the United States.

Further research into the tolcapone database created from the Medline articles revealed that one of the most recent articles on the topic included a 2007 article documenting a study examining the efficacy and safety of replacing entacapone (another anti-Parkinson's pharmaceutical) with tolcapone in Parkinson's disease patients. The authors, cited as "The Entacapone to

Tolcapone Switch Study Investigators," similarly comprised of 30 separate centers and investigators, concluded that "there was a tendency for tolcapone to offer enhanced efficacy in patients with fluctuating Parkinson's disease, despite optimized entacapone therapy. Tolcapone can be considered, therefore, for patients whose motor fluctuations are inadequately controlled by their existing regimen" (The Entacapone to Tolcapone Switch Study Investigators, 2007, p. 14). The acknowledgements in the article stated that the study was sponsored by Hoffmann-La Roche Laboratories. As tolcapone was withdrawn in Canada 9 years earlier yet remains on the market alongside entacapone in the United States and Europe, the study was most likely aimed at physicians prescribing in the United States and Europe and perhaps increasingly choosing entacapone to treat their Parkinson's patients. After all, an influential study published in 2000 in the journal *Neurology* stated that

> although the benefits observed with tolcapone were comparable to, or slightly better than those observed with entacapone, tolcapone had been restricted to use in patients who failed to respond to other adjunctive agents, required more frequent and restrictive liver blood test monitoring and had been removed from the market in other countries [due to hepatic problems]. Conversely, no hepatic problems have been encountered with entacapone. (Kieburtz & Hubble, 2000, S45)

Despite the influence of the Internet on patients' knowledge about and requests for prescription medications (Mintzes et al., 2002), "most patients remain significantly dependent on their physicians for knowledge about their prescription medicines" (Abraham & Davis, 2007, p. 418). Physicians are, in turn, dependent on the information approved by the regulatory authorities (most often found in the pharmaceutical information pamphlet), as well as scientific publications, for their knowledge about the pharmaceuticals that they are prescribing. In the meantime, regulatory officials depend on pharmaceutical manufacturers for results of tests and trials in order to make their risk–benefit assessments (Abraham & Davis, 2007). Unfortunately, all of these expectations rest on manufacturers who possess a biased interest when assimilating scientific information into the contents of the pharmaceutical's monograph or related publications.

5.3. THE ROLE OF USER FEES

In addition to the manipulation of scientific and medical literature, there exists substantial evidence that those scrutinizing pharmaceuticals for approval have also been "contaminated" by the seemingly far-reaching tentacles of pharmaceutical manufacturers. Market-driven concerns about patent life, profitability, and investor stock prices provide strong incentives for these behaviors (Petersen, 2000). The development of new pharmaceuticals is an enormous undertaking involving thousands of people and hundreds of millions of dollars, demonstrating that finances serve as a major actor involved in pharmaceutical networks, and as a result, strongly influence the practices of other networked actors. It can be concluded that the pharmaceutical companies want the safety and efficacy standards of regulators to be high enough to avoid frequent "pharmaceutical disasters" that bring the industry into disrepute, but not so high that they threaten their commercial viability (Abraham, 2002a, p. 1498). For example, a manufacturer can lose on average over US$1 million for each day's delay in gaining marketing approval from the FDA (Montaner, O'Shaughnessy, & Schechter, 2001). As a result, when governments become involved in the regulation of the pharmaceutical industry, presumably on behalf of patients' interests in the safety and effectiveness of pharmaceuticals, the pharmaceutical industry is no longer seen simply as a commercial entity but rather becomes a "political player focused on influencing the principles and processes defining regulation" (Abraham, 2002b, p. 1498). Evidence shows that interactions with industry pose a serious threat to the public's health interests, and in the case of health research and the field of medicine, such interaction jeopardizes medical ethics and patient interests at the expense of satisfying private interests (Mather, 2005). In 1981 John McKinlay asserted that "the claims of manufacturers, opinions of enthusiastic researchers, the well-intentioned adoption by experienced clinicians and educators, as well as public demand, are no substitute for a proper evaluation, and do not provide a rational scientific basis for policy decisions" (p. 386). This comment is as poignant today, perhaps even more so, as it was when written by McKinlay over two decades ago.

Anecdotal evidence suggests that conflicts of interest with pharmaceutical manufacturers can affect a committee vote (Lurie, 2006). In 2005 the FDA convened a meeting to discuss the toxicity of cyclooxygenase-II enzyme (COX-2; an enzyme responsible for inflammation and pain) inhibitors Celebrex® and Bextra®, both multimillion dollar[2] pain relievers developed to be gentler on the stomach than other, older pain relievers. The meeting was held in response to manufacturer Merck voluntarily withdrawing Vioxx from the market in September of 2004 amid safety concerns (Steinbrook, 2005). Had the committee members with ties to industry been precluded from voting at the meeting discussing the future of COX-2 inhibitors, the committee would more than likely have voted against the return of Vioxx and the continued approval of Celebrex and Bextra; but instead, all three pharmaceuticals received favorable votes (Harris & Berenson, 2005). In a subsequent highly publicized study, FDA drug researcher Dr. David Graham and colleagues found a four-fold increase in cardiovascular risk in patients using this class of drugs compared to others, resulting in "an estimated 88,000 to 140,000 excess cases of serious coronary heart disease" from COX-2 inhibitors (Graham et al., 2005, p. 480). Lurie, Almeida, Stine, Stine, and Wolfe (2006) published a study in the *Journal of the American Medical Association* that examined the prevalence and consequences of financial conflicts at these meetings over 4 years. At least one advisory committee member had a financial link to the pharmaceutical's maker or a competitor in 73% of meetings. Those committee members with disclosed conflicts were 10% more likely to favor the pharmaceutical being considered.

Lurie et al.'s (2006) findings suggest that in today's climate, the committees considering the approval and withdrawal of both pemoline and tolcapone were likely influenced by the manufacturers in some way. While evidence in the cases of pemoline and tolcapone was unavailable regarding committee members' names or conflicts of interest, it appears to me that this was entirely likely, especially in the case of pemoline which was approved in the 1970s, long before any requirements precluding those with conflict of interests or their disclosure were put in place. Although it could be argued that the pharmaceutical industry was not as sophisticated in influencing officials then, it is nonetheless highly unlikely that no exchanges occurred at all. In addition, although I do not have any evidence in the form of specific examples of pharmaceutical industry tampering or provision of financial incentives for favorable regulatory outcomes, I suspect that it took place if only for the reasons that it took over 20 years for the withdrawal of pemoline off the Canadian market and over 30 years in the United States. With such serious adverse effects known from the initial stages of preapproval, as well as other safer pharmaceuticals available for treatment of the same condition, one would assume that the pharmaceutical would have been withdrawn long before it had been. In addition, the FDA did not actively withdraw the pharmaceutical, but rather was pressured by Public Citizen to do so, and only then did the manufacturers themselves stop production ahead of any official FDA withdrawal.

With regard to tolcapone, the fact that the FDA approved the pharmaceutical for sale after numerous patient deaths and withdrawals in other countries appears questionable. As mentioned previously, it was being approved in the United States at the same time that it was "on its way out" in Canada. In addition, its very lengthy series of serious patient adverse effects and warnings makes one question whether its single benefit did, indeed, outweigh its many safety risks. One obvious example of pharmaceutical company prowess in governmental regulation is that of lobbyists. Both Canadian and American pharmaceutical manufacturers fund strong lobbying groups to persuade government officials' decision making. According to the Center for Responsive Politics in the United States, a nonpartisan, independent, and nonprofit organization dedicated to the analysis and dissemination of political campaign contributions and lobbying data, "[T]he pharmaceutical manufacturing industry has had one of the largest lobbying efforts on Capitol Hill for years. Top lobbyists include PhRMA, Pfizer, and Amgen Inc., with lobbying efforts focusing on patent reform, research funding and Medicare" (Center for Responsive Politics, 2008). In the 2008 election cycle, for example, the top 20 pharmaceutical manufacturers' contributions to federal candidates and parties totaled almost US$8 million while in 2007, the total amount spent on lobbying was US$150 million (Center for Responsive Politics, 2008). Although the lobbying efforts in the cases of pemoline and tolcapone are unquantifiable, they serve as other very likely actors in the networks of both pharmaceuticals because both manufacturers are aware of the concept. In 2008, for example, Abbott Laboratories, the manufacturer of pemoline, spent US$880,000, while Hoffmann-La Roche spent US$1,712,417 (Center for Responsive Politics, 2008).

As we know, since the early- to mid-1990s, pharmaceutical companies have paid user fees for a variety of pharmaceutical approval-related activities carried out by the Therapeutic Products Directorate in Canada. In his study exploring whether changes in approval times for new active substances coincided with the level of user fees, Lexchin (2006b) collected data from a range of Canadian government publications on the following topics: total funding for and workload of the regulatory agencies, the percentage of income that came from tax revenue and user fees, the percentage of new pharmaceutical submissions that received a positive decision, and the percent of submissions that were approved on first review. What he found was a moderate-to-strong positive association between the level of industry funding and the percent of submissions that received a positive decision and a moderate-to-strong negative association between the level of industry funding and approval times. In effect, this creates a situation favorable to the pharmaceutical industry.

Three opinion articles, issued by the *New England Journal of Medicine* in April of 2007, argued that the scheme wherein manufacturers fund agencies responsible for approving their products results in a conflict of interest for both U.S. and Canadian governing bodies and worries physicians and academics alike. Jerry Avorn, a professor of medicine at Harvard, asserted that the FDA is unique in that it is the only regulatory agency that works "so cosily" with a trade group that represents the industry, in this case the Pharmaceutical Research and Manufacturers of America (PhRMA; 2007, p. 1698). In his article, Avorn called for Congress to sever this relationship by requiring that "the FDA's pharmaceutical-related work...be funded by general federal revenues, rather than by the industry it regulates" (Avorn, p. 1700).

> Most federal regulatory agencies do not derive such a large proportion of their operating budgets from the industries that they oversee, nor is it typical for such relationships to be negotiated so closely between government and the trade groups representing the industry. (Avorn, p. 1700)

Yet the current FDA proposal for the renewal of the Prescription Drug User Fee Act (PDUFA) was developed along with PhRMA, as was Canada's Research-Based Pharmaceutical Companies' goals adoption by the Therapeutic Products Directorate (Lexchin, 2006b). No similar influence has been exerted by any other industry on a government agency, making the public question the FDA's integrity (Thompson, 2000). Under the arrangement in the United States, the safety considerations and risks of pharmaceuticals already approved for marketing are not examined routinely nor in significant amounts due to the fact that the FDA possesses very limited resources in order to conduct postmarketing pharmaceutical safety testing. For instance, one article pointed out that the 5% of the user fees permitted to go to postmarketing safety testing is not enough for the FDA to conduct "even a single large study of one recently noted safety signal that has major public health importance—the indication of possible cardiovascular risk posed by pharmaceuticals for attention deficit-hyperactivity disorder" (Hennessy & Strom, 2007, p. 1703).

In the United States, opposition to current pharmaceutical safety legislation is growing, as a group of 22 experts on pharmaceutical safety and regulation, and a coalition of 12 patient, consumer, science, and public health organizations issued two separate open letters to lawmakers in 2007. The letter from the safety and regulation experts called for lawmakers to "not reauthorize the user fees system that finances the review of new pharmaceuticals by the Food and Drug Administration" (Wood, 2007). "User fees may appear to save the taxpayer money, but at an unacceptable cost to public health," the letter warned, citing findings of a panel of experts recently convened by the Institute of Medicine (IOM) to address pharmaceutical safety at the FDA (Wood). The letter called for Congress to "reassess the system in which pharmaceuticals are developed, tested, approved and followed post-approval, with support for replacing the current user fee model with increased direct funding for the FDA" (Wood). The letter was signed by pharmaceutical safety expert Dr. Jerome Avorn; four IOM panel members, including Dr. Bruce Psaty and Professor Alta Charo; three former editors-in-chief of the *New England Journal of Medicine*, Dr. Marcia Angell, Dr. Jerome Kassirer, and Dr. Arnold Relman; and former assistant secretary for public health Phil Lee, along with other respected experts from the medical, academic, and public policy fields.

The letter from the coalition of patient, consumer, science, and public health organizations agreed that PDUFA is undermining patient safety, stating that it "does not include the provisions necessary to prevent another Vioxx, Accutane[3], or Ketek from reaching the market and harming patients and their families" (Miller, 2007). Both letters cited the need for reforms suggested by the IOM panel, which found that the "FDA's pharmaceutical safety system is impaired by resource constraints, problems with organizational culture, and unclear and insufficient regulatory authority" (Miller).

Recommendations contained in the 22 experts' letter included the elimination of deadlines or targets for speed of review in order to allow flexibility and adequate time for evaluation and analysis by reviewers; the setting of new performance goals linked with safety or other public health outcomes, not just quick approval decisions; as well as the ensuring that sufficient resources are available for scientific research and training for FDA staff. All signers of both letters agreed that "The FDA's mission is to protect and advance the public's health. As it currently exists, and would exist in its proposed form, PDUFA stands in the way of this objective" (Wood, 2007).

One could argue that the speeding up of approval times for pharmaceuticals, through additional funding from the pharmaceutical industry, could allow patients to access much needed drugs such as anti-AIDS medications sooner than traditional regulations would permit. According to Abraham (2002a, p. 1166), however, evidence to support this hypothesis is scarce compared with the amount of evidence stating that quicker pharmaceutical approval times have been a result of making regulatory agencies more responsive to the profit-making interests of the pharmaceutical industry. In addition, if the speeding up of approval times for new pharmaceuticals was truly driven by the need to provide faster access to new treatments, an associated initiation of regulatory requirements requiring comparisons of efficacy of new compounds with existing ones would be put in place in order to demonstrate that a new pharmaceutical does indeed offer a genuine advancement over existing treatments. However, neither the European Commission nor the governments of the European Union, North America, or Japan have introduced such requirements (Abraham, 2002a, p. 1166). In addition, evidence is accumulating that the emphasis on speedy approvals may lead to problematic decision making. Data analyzed by

Daniel Carpenter, a professor of government policy at Harvard University, suggest that pharmaceuticals approved just before the PDUFA deadlines are far more likely to cause safety problems after they are in widespread use than those approved at other points in the review cycle (Carpenter, Zucker, & Avorn, 2008). Neither pemoline (which was approved before the PDUFA came into effect) nor tolcapone (which took 19 months to approve due to five separate resubmissions being requested of the manufacturer by the FDA) were approved by the PDUFA deadlines.

5.4. THE ROLE OF PHYSICIANS IN MARKETING PRACTICES

Although pharmaceutical companies are investing large amounts of resources into ensuring that their products are approved for sale, they are also spending increasing amounts convincing physicians to prescribe their products: During the first 9 months of 1998, US$2.7 billion was spent on sales and promotional efforts to office-based physicians (Maguire, 1999). It is no secret that pharmaceutical manufacturers, as others in industries involved in the development of products, often fund physicians and researchers, as well as their projects, symposia, and certain professional gatherings (Lexchin, 1984; Loe, 2004; Mather, 2005). In return, certain physicians "moonlight as consultants" for these companies (Stipp & Moore, 1998, p. 120). Experts and marketers are progressively more dependent on each other since experts require funding for their research and marketers require expert support in order to exude authority and to publish data on pharmaceuticals. This arrangement constitutes a large portion of the modern medical landscape (Loe, 2004). Katherine Greider, author of the book entitled *The Big Fix: How the Pharmaceutical Industry Rips off American Consumers*, wrote that this fusion of science and capitalism has left the United States (as can be assumed for Canada as well) "oddly impoverished in the way of unbiased, approachable information about the usefulness and cost of one pharmaceutical versus another" (2003, p. 2). Undoubtedly, the situation calls into effect Moynihan and Cassels' (2005) assertion that "a medical profession too inebriated by the largesse of profit-driven pharmaceutical companies cannot serve the public interest" (p. viii).

According to pharmaceutical company income statements, pharmaceutical makers generally spend twice as much to market pharmaceuticals as they do to research them (Harris, 2007). Hence, despite limited knowledge about the safety of a new pharmaceutical, it may be approved, readily prescribed by physicians, and purchased by patients. Pharmaceutical companies often actively promote early use of new pharmaceuticals and seek to influence physicians and patients through direct-to-consumer marketing in order to rapidly increase sales and form prescribing patterns ahead of competitors (Basara, 1996; Jones, Greenfield, & Bradley, 2001; Peay & Peay, 1988; Stross, 1987). Direct-to-consumer pharmaceutical advertising, although often containing misleading claims and lacking risk-related information (Department of Health and Human Services, 1998a, 2001), also generates a high volume of new pharmaceutical prescriptions (Basara, 1996).

Regarding the pharmaceuticals in question in this study, direct-to-consumer promotional materials were distributed by Hoffmann-La Roche in order to market Tasmar. According to two letters to the manufacturer I obtained from the FDA, these materials were found to be in violation of the Federal Food, Pharmaceutical, and Cosmetic Act and applicable regulations in the United States because they contained misleading claims and lacked risk-related information. The materials in question included "physician starter packs, bottle holders and packers" (Department of Health and Human Services, n.d., p. 1) and a "Coming Soon" advertisement in the September 1997 issue of *Archives of Neurology and Neurology Reviews* (Department of Health and Human Services, 1998a). Specifically, the Division of Pharmaceutical Marketing, Advertising, and Communications of the FDA objected to the fact that there were misleading claims in the starter packs, bottle holders, and packers because the manufacturer employed three prohibited claims. The first was "Introducing…" which was deemed to be misleading because at the time of distribution of the materials, Tasmar was not a new pharmaceutical and its introduction period was over. The second and third were "the first and only COMT inhibitor" and "completely new kind…" respectively. These statements were deemed to be unacceptable because "a new COMT inhibitor was approved in October of 1999, [so] Tasmar was not the only COMT inhibitor." Similarly, Tasmar was not a "completely new kind of treatment for Parkinson's Disease" (Department of Health and Human Services, n.d., p. 1). The letter also cited a "lack of fair balance" in the cited Tasmar promotional materials because they had "insufficient risk information to balance the claims about the pharmaceutical." The letter continued that "Tasmar is a second line pharmaceutical for Parkinson's disease, and has a boxed warning about the risk of fatal, acute fulminant liver failure and the need for patient monitoring. This important risk information is not presented in the materials" (Department of Health and Human Services, n.d., p. 2). In addition, "[the statement] as with all pharmaceuticals, side effects may occur with Tasmar is not adequate as fair balance and minimizes the risks associated with Tasmar" (Department of Health and Human Services, n.d., p. 2). Furthermore, the manufacturer had not submitted these promotional materials to the appropriate agency for review of labeling and advertising prior to the time of initial distribution, a requirement of the department.

The "Coming Soon" advertisement in the September 1997 issue of *Archives of Neurology and Neurology Reviews* warranted a letter from the Division of Pharmaceutical Marketing, Advertising, and Communications because the claims in the advertisement constituted preapproval promotion of Tasmar. The letter noted that "the Code of Federal Regulations states that a sponsor...shall not represent in a promotional context that an investigational pharmaceutical is safe or effective for the purposes for which it is under investigation or otherwise promote the pharmaceutical" (Department of Health and Human Services, 1998a, p. 1). Allowable "Coming Soon" advertisements are permitted to announce the name of the product without making any written, verbal, or graphic representations about its safety, efficacy, or intended use (p. 1). The advertisement in question, however,

> [made] several representations about the product's intended use and its mechanism of action. Tasmar [would] be the first and only COMT inhibitor indicated for Parkinson's disease. Thus, the graphic presentation of the inhibition of COMT, both in the flow chart and in the pharmacokinetics profile [made] a product-specific representation about Tasmar. (Department of Health and Human Services, 1998a, p. 1)

Further, the claim that an "important new development in levodopa metabolism" was "coming soon from Roche" was also a product-specific representation of Tasmar (p. 2). Finally, if there could be any doubt that the pharmaceutical product in question was intended for use in therapy for Parkinson's disease, "this advertisement was a derivative of a current full product advertisement that Roche used for levodopa tablets" (p. 2). Both letters requested that the manufacturer immediately stop further dissemination of the stated products and advertisements and respond, in writing, with its intent to comply. With regards to advertising for pemoline, Freeman (1976, p. 10) stated that Abbott Laboratories placed "glowing reports and advertising" for pemoline in many medical journals during 1975, although these could not be found.

Pharmaceutical companies claim that "direct-to-consumer advertising has an educational function that creates better informed consumers, encouraging them to consult their physicians about underdiagnosed symptoms and treatment options" and allowing patients to make better health care choices (Lyles, 2002, as cited in Conrad & Leiter, 2004, p. 161; see also Bonaccorso & Sturchio, 2002). The American College of Physicians, however, has stated its position that consumer advertising "does not constitute appropriate patient education" (Maguire, 1999). Regardless, 3.5% of Canadian patients and 8.2% of U.S. patients report using advertising as an information source (Mintzes et al., 2002). Although these figures appear negligible, it must be considered that although some patients may not consciously employ such sources to provide information, they nonetheless internalize the messages they are exposed to daily by various media.

The study by Mintzes et al. (2002) compared prescribing decisions in a U.S. setting with legal direct-to-consumer advertising and a Canadian setting where such advertising of prescription pharmaceuticals is illegal but where some cross-border exposure occurs. The results suggest that more advertising leads to more requests for advertised medicines and more prescriptions. If direct-to-consumer advertising opens a conversation between patients and physicians, that conversation is highly likely to end with a prescription, often despite physician ambivalence about treatment choice. According to Mintzes et al., physicians fulfilled, on average, 75% of requests for direct-to-consumer advertised pharmaceuticals (2002). Conrad and Leiter hypothesized that in this way, pharmaceutical manufacturers are circumventing physicians' control over knowledge regarding available pharmaceuticals (2004).

Physicians are increasingly frustrated that the developments associated with increased direct-to-patient advertising are putting their patients in the "diagnostic driver's seat" (Maguire, 1999). Some note that increasingly, patients are presenting them with lists of pharmaceuticals which they would like to try, many of which are neither "time-tested" nor "cost effective" (Maguire, 1999). Other physicians state that patients believe that certain (advertised) pharmaceuticals are going to be a panacea for their problems, and as a result, pressure the physicians for prescriptions, regardless if the physician feels otherwise. It must be noted, however, that these sentiments rely on the belief that physicians are selfless workers on the patient's behalf who only do what is necessary for them, including prescribing only time-tested and cost-effective medications. This is not always true, however, as is evidenced by the biases incurred by physicians who take part in, or themselves organize, promotional efforts, consultations, and symposia on behalf of pharmaceutical manufacturers (Lexchin, 1984; Loe, 2004; Maguire, 1999; Mather, 2005; Stipp & Moore, 1998).

As can be gleaned from the aforementioned marketing practices of the manufacturer, new pharmaceutical products are often advertised even before they are available for public use. Pharmaceutical firms may rush new pharmaceuticals to market because of concerns about patent life, a desire to mould prescribing habits prior to the market entry of competitions, and hopes for a fast "ramp-up" in sales that will encourage investors and increase stock prices (Hurwitz & Caves, 1988; Murphy, Smith, & Juergens, 1992). While the previous examples relate to advertising aimed at medical professionals, I also searched for, but was not able to find, advertisements for pemoline and tolcapone aimed at the general public. Perhaps I could not find these sources for a few reasons: First, pemoline was approved for use in Canada and the United States in the late 1970s, before any direct-to-consumer advertising was permitted in Canada or the United States.[4] In addition, although this form of advertising gained approval from the FDA by late 1985 in the United States, manufacturers overwhelmingly chose to advertise prescription medications in television commercials rather than print ads, the former of which were not accessible to me. Although the popularity of print advertisements for prescription pharmaceuticals gained momentum throughout the 1990s, I found no advertisements for pemoline. Regarding tolcapone, although it was approved in the late 1990s, there were no print advertisements aimed at the general public. This may be because it is an adjunct to a very specific treatment affecting a relatively small population of patients, in which case advertising would likely be more beneficial in the form of direct-to-physician materials.

5.5. FAILURE OF THE BLACK BOX—
ADVERSE REACTION REPORTS

> *Adverse drug reactions are believed to be a leading cause of death in the United Sates.*
> —Lazarou, Pomeranz, and Corey (1998, p. 1200)

Before a pharmaceutical product is placed on the market, known information on its safety and efficacy is limited, regardless of the number of journal articles published on it. This stems from the fact that relatively few patients participate in clinical trials compared with the number of users required to detect uncommon adverse reactions (Colosimo, 1999). In addition, clinical trial participants are a select and homogeneous group of individuals that meet specific criteria (Brewer & Colditz, 1999). Clinical trials are, therefore, not necessarily representative of the "real world" and the real degree of risk to users is not always known. "In evaluating pharmaceuticals for approval," Friedman and colleagues note that the FDA (like Heath Canada) "uses a pragmatic standard: do the demonstrated benefits outweigh the known risks?" (Friedman et al., 1999, p. 1732). Clearly, this is not nearly as easy or neat as plugging terms into an equation—how can one ever turn the effects of pharmaceuticals into measureable terms for an equation? Obviously, there is a lot of debate and struggle among reviewers over what are deemed to be "benefits" and "risks." Nevertheless, all of this debate appears to be glossed over after the fact of approval.

Regarding the pharmaceuticals in question, the reviewer documents associated with the approval of tolcapone in the United States serve as a robust example of the frailty of the equation upon which approval rests. In his recommendation letter, reviewer Dr. Russell Katz wrote,

> The sponsor has submitted sufficient information to permit a conclusion that tolcapone is effective as an adjunctive treatment to levodopa/carbidopa for Parkinson's disease patients with or without end of dose wearing off phenomena. In addition, the sponsor has submitted *sufficient safety information to permit a preliminary conclusion that tolcapone is acceptably safe* [italics added]...for these reasons, I recommend that the sponsor be sent the attached Approvable Letter. (Division of Neuropharmacological Pharmaceutical Products—Food and Drug Administration, 1997)

The aforementioned sentence states that "sufficient" safety information allows reviewers to permit "preliminary" conclusions that the pharmaceutical in question is "acceptably safe."

All of these terms point to a lack of compelling and persuasive decision making. Rather, the decision appears to be made based largely on overstated conclusions and language.

At the time of tolcapone's approval in both Canada and the United States, the pharmaceutical's risks, especially those of hepatotoxicity, were well-known despite a lack of sufficient knowledge as to why they occurred. Nonetheless, the pharmaceutical was approved provided that these precautions and adverse reactions were printed on its product monograph as well as a patient consent form being signed by individual patients in front of their prescribing physicians. Among the statements contained on the consent form were the following:

> "I understand that there is a serious risk that I could develop severe liver failure, which may be potentially fatal, by using Tasmar."

> "I understand that there are no laboratory tests that will predict if I am at an increased risk for fatal liver failure."

> "I understand that although blood work may help detect if I develop liver failure it may do so only after significant, irreversible and potentially fatal damage has already occurred."

> "I understand that I must immediately report any unusual symptoms to my doctor." (Tasmar Product Monograph, 1998)

The precautions found on the 1998 version of the product monograph in the United States included the following black box warning:

> Because of the risk of potentially fatal, acute fulminant liver failure, TASMAR (tolcapone) should ordinarily be used in patients with Parkinson's disease on levodopa / carbidopa who are experiencing symptom fluctuations and are

not responding satisfactorily to or are not appropriate candidates for other adjunctive therapies. Because of the risk of liver injury and because TASMAR, when it is effective, provides an observable symptomatic benefit, the patient who fails to show substantial clinical benefit within 3 weeks of initiation of treatment, should be withdrawn from TASMAR…Cases of severe hepatocellular injury, including fulminant liver failure resulting in death, have been reported in post-marketing use. As of October 1998, 3 cases of fatal fulminant hepatic failure have been reported from approximately 60,000 patients providing about 40,000 patient years of worldwide use. This incidence may be 10- to 100- fold higher than the background incidence in the general population. Underreporting of cases may lead to significant underestimation of the increased risk associated with the use of TASMAR…Although a program of frequent laboratory monitoring for evidence of hepatocellular injury is deemed essential, it is not clear that baseline and periodic monitoring of liver enzymes will prevent the occurrence of fulminant liver failure. (Tasmar Product Monograph, 1998, p. 1)

Furthermore, about half of the 23 pages of the product monograph are dedicated solely to disclosing and warning against other serious adverse reactions caused by the drug. These included 57 different adverse reactions experienced by a minimum of 1% of the 298 clinical trial participants with Parkinson's disease (malaise, panic reaction, tumor of the skin, cataracts, euphoria, fever, alopecia, eye inflammation, hypertonia, and tumor of the uterus) up to a maximum of 51% (dyskinesia[5]). Furthermore, other adverse reactions which were observed during all trials in patients with Parkinson's disease included the following, grouped into respective body systems:

> *Nervous System—frequent*: depression, hyperesthesia, tremor, speech disorder, vertigo, emotional lability; *infrequent*: neuralgia, amnesia, extrapyramidal syndrome,

hostility, libido increased, manic reaction, nervousness, paranoid reaction, cerebral ischemia, cerebrovascular accident, delusions, libido decreased, neuropathy, apathy, choreoathetosis, myoclonus, psychosis, thinking abnormal, twitching; *rare*: antisocial reaction, delirium, encephalopathy, hemiplegia, meningitis.

Digestive System—frequent: tooth disorder; *infrequent*: dysphagia, gastrointestinal hemorrhage, gastroenteritis, mouth ulceration, increased salivation, abnormal stools, esophagitis, cholelithiasis, colitis, tongue disorder, rectal disorder; *rare*: cholecystitis, duodenal ulcer, gastrointestinal carcinoma, stomach atony.

Body as a Whole—frequent: flank pain, accidental injury, abdominal pain, infection; *infrequent*: hernia, pain, allergic reaction, cellulitis, infection fungal, viral infection, carcinoma, chills, infection bacterial, neoplasm, abscess, face edema; *rare*: death.

Cardiovascular System—frequent: palpitation; *infrequent*: hypertension, vasodilation, angina pectoris, heart failure, atrial fibrillation, tachycardia, migraine, aortic stenosis, arrhythmia, arteriospasm, bradycardia, cerebral hemorrhage, coronary artery disorder, heart arrest, myocardial infarct, myocardial ischemia, pulmonary embolus; *rare*: arteriosclerosis, cardiovascular disorder, pericardial effusion, thrombosis.

Musculoskeletal System—frequent: myalgia; *infrequent*: tenosynovitis, arthrosis, joint disorder.

Urogenital System—frequent: urinary incontinence, impotence; *infrequent*: prostatic disorder, dysuria, nocturia, polyuria, urinary retention, urinary tract disorder, hematuria, kidney calculus, prostatic carcinoma, breast neoplasm, oliguria, uterine atony, uterine disorder, vaginitis;

rare: bladder calculus, ovarian carcinoma, uterine hemorrhage.

Respiratory System—frequent: bronchitis, pharyngitis; *infrequent*: cough increased, rhinitis, asthma, epistaxis, hyperventilation, laryngitis, hiccup; *rare*: apnea, hypoxia, lung edema.

Skin and Appendages—frequent: rash; *infrequent*: herpes zoster, pruritus, seborrhea, skin discoloration, eczema, erythema multiforme, skin disorder, furunculosis, herpes simplex, urticaria.

Special Senses—frequent: tinnitus; *infrequent*: diplopia, ear pain, eye hemorrhage, eye pain, lacrimation disorder, otitis media, parosmia; *rare*: glaucoma.

Metabolic and Nutritional—infrequent: edema, hypercholesteremia, thirst, dehydration.

Hemic and Lymphatic System—infrequent: anemia; *rare:* leukemia, thrombocytopenia.

Endocrine System—infrequent: diabetes mellitus. (Tasmar Product Monograph, 1998, p. 19)

Similarly to tolcapone's case, at the time of pemoline's approval in the United States, there also remained multiple safety issues and adverse reactions caused by the pharmaceutical which had not been sufficiently studied to warrant concrete knowledge of its workings. Nonetheless, the pharmaceutical was approved provided that these precautions and adverse reactions were printed on its product monograph (Food and Drug Administration, 1974). These precautions included the following statements found on the product monograph in the United States:

—"The interaction of Cylert with other pharmaceuticals has not been studied in humans."

—"Data are not available concerning long term effects on mutagenicity in animals or humans."

—"There are no adequate and well-controlled studies in pregnant women."

—"Studies in rats have shown an increased incidence of stillbirths and cannibalization when pemoline was administered."

—"Safety and effectiveness in children below the age of 5 years have not been established. Long-term effects of Cylert in children have not been established."

—"Central nervous system stimulants, including pemoline, have been reported to precipitate motor and phonic tics and Tourette's syndrome."

—"There have been reports of hepatic dysfunction including elevated liver enzymes, hepatitis and jaundice in patients taking Cylert. The occurrence of elevated liver enzymes is not rare and these reactions appear to be reversible upon pharmaceutical discontinuance. Most patients with elevated liver enzymes were asymptomatic. Although no causal relationship has been established, two hepatic-related fatalities have been reported involving patients taking Cylert."

—"Literature reports indicate that Cylert may precipitate attacks of Gilles de la Tourette syndrome: hallucinations, dyskinetic movements of the tongue, lips, face and extremities; abnormal oculomotor function...mild depression, dizziness, increasing irritability, headache and drowsiness...anorexia and weight loss...nausea and stomach ache...skin rash." (Cylert Product Monograph, 1984, p. 5)

As can be clearly seen from the combination of the patient consent form, black box warning, and documented adverse reactions in preapproval clinical trials, both pemoline and tolcapone could certainly be considered risky and potentially problematic when administered. However, a larger number of patients were nonetheless willing to bear the risk of all of the potential adverse reactions with the hope that these medications would improve the symptoms of either ADHD or Parkinson's disease. Although we do not know the exact criteria employed by Health Canada and the FDA in approving these pharmaceuticals, we do know that these were dependent on the pharmaceuticals themselves and focused on their risks versus their benefits. During the approval process, the regulatory agencies' actions served to illustrate the belief that pemoline's benefit of once-a-day dosing overshadowed its many possible risks, while for tolcapone, the potential benefit of prolonged "on times" for Parkinson's disease patients outweighed the many serious risks in the hypothetical risk–benefit equation. After all, these were repeatedly stated as the major benefits of these pharmaceuticals over other existing ones and served as the major reasons for their approval. Looking back, it appears foolish that what appear to be relatively superficial benefits served to overshadow all of the serious risks posed by these pharmaceuticals, so much so that they warranted approval and, as a result, caused numerous patient deaths and serious injuries for years to come. As a result, it appears that the entire networks around both of these pharmaceuticals were stabilized, if only briefly, in the absence of what we normally think of as medical benefits, resulting in both pemoline and tolcapone being seen and employed as bona fide pharmaceuticals tested and keenly approved to help patients.

As can been seen from the cases of pemoline and tolcapone, at the time of regulatory approval for most pharmaceuticals, a number of issues remain unknown: the occurrence of rare but serious adverse events, pharmaceutical interactions, adverse events during treatment or after the discontinuation of treatment, effects in pregnancy, or differential effects in subgroups that may be defined by age, sex, or race. Nonetheless, both manufacturers and approval agencies tend to believe that the natural history of prescription pharmaceuticals, after approval, includes the accumulation of new information on risks and benefits because regulatory approval for clinical use "does not and cannot guarantee safety" (Gale, 2001, p. 1871). In effect, all (or arguably, most) information on a pharmaceutical cannot be known prior to approval, and so it is discovered with extended use by patients. Unfortunately, the existence of such evidence as a pharmaceutical's link to serious adverse events in patients appears to be dependent on the number of patient years (number of patients taking the pharmaceutical multiplied by the duration of doses taken) of experience with a pharmaceutical, which undoubtedly allows for an increased amount of risk to patients taking a relatively new, understudied compound. Nonetheless, in some cases, approvals have been granted even when serious adverse pharmaceutical reactions were detected by premarketing clinical trials; for example, the nighttime heartburn pharmaceutical Propulsid® was found to cause heart-rhythm disorders (Willman, 2000). In the cases of both pemoline and tolcapone, serious or even fatal liver failure did not prevent approval of either.

The *Physicians' Desk Reference*, an annual compendium of the FDA-approved professional product labeling for selected pharmaceuticals, is released each November. Black box warnings, such as that found for tolcapone, are prominently displayed in the publication in order to alert practitioners to serious health risks associated with certain pharmaceuticals (Beach, Faich, Bormel, & Sasinowski, 1998). According to the *Federal Register* (1998, as cited in Lasser et al., 2002),

[S]pecial problems, particularly those that may lead to death or serious injury, may be required by the Food and Drug Administration to be placed in a prominently displayed box. The boxed warning ordinarily shall be based on clinical data, but serious animal toxicity may also be the basis of a boxed warning in the absence of clinical data.

Lasser et al. (2002) recently reported that of 548 new pharmaceuticals approved by the FDA between 1975 and 1999, 56 (10.2%) acquired a black box warning (such as tolcapone) and 16 (2.9%) were withdrawn from the market. This translates into a 20% probability of a new pharmaceutical acquiring a black box warning or being withdrawn from the market over a 25-year period. Half of these warnings and withdrawals occurred within 7 years of the pharmaceutical's introduction, and half of the withdrawals occurred within 2 years, a finding consistent with previous research (Bakke, Manocchia, de Abajo, Kaitin, & Lasagna, 1995). These data show that serious adverse pharmaceutical reactions occurring after governmental agency approval has been granted are not uncommon and should be a cause for concern.

The functions of pharmaceutical regulation include regulation both before and after sales approval; however, in practice, approval for sale has been the most important form of public regulation on pharmaceuticals (Abraham & Lawton Smith, 2003). In the Description chapter, I provided a detailed examination of the pharmaceutical approval processes for both Canada and the United States. There are no precise preclinical or clinical data requirements for pharmaceuticals in Canada or the United States. In fact, a spokeswoman for Health Canada has noted that "Health Canada does not have a set policy on how long or how many people a company has to test a pharmaceutical. In general, they say this varies with the disease and the expected outcome" (Skerritt, 2007, p. A2).

In order to better acquaint myself with the issues surrounding approval and withdrawal of both pemoline and tolcapone in Canada, I contacted Health Canada with a Freedom of Information Act request to see any documents which were available concerning the decision-making processes surrounding both pemoline and tolcapone approval and/or withdrawal. Although I requested the documentation in August of 2007, by the time of the printing of this book, nothing had yet been delivered. Of course, dozens of telephone calls and e-mails were sent to respective personnel, but to no avail. Each time, I was told that the requested documents were going to be sent out "soon" pending approval from a certain department and/or "third party." By May of 2008, Health Canada notified me that it was willing to send me more information on its decision to approve Cylert, yet "privacy concerns" were cited by the manufacturer and these documents could not be delivered to me, pending an appeal on my behalf. In the end, Health Canada did not send anything, although I suspect that having the documents would not have clarified much regarding each pharmaceutical's risk–benefit equation for approval and withdrawal, as it seems to me that Health Canada does not have a clear formula for each pharmaceutical's equation.

It can be concluded that, generally, once a pharmaceutical is approved for sale on the market, it is "black boxed" in ANT terms, and everything is assumed to be in adequate order by the general public regarding the pharmaceutical's safety. Furthermore, much of the information provided about the pharmaceutical by national regulatory agencies or pharmaceutical manufacturers is considered to be "scientific" and based on tried and tested "facts" and as such, trusted by millions of individuals making important decisions about their health care. As Susan Leigh Star (1991, as cited in John Law, 1991) wrote,

> A fact is born in a laboratory, becomes stripped of its contingency and the process of its production to appear in its facticity as Truth. Some Truths and technologies, joined in networks of translation, become enormously stable features of our landscape, shaping action and inhibiting certain kinds of change. (p. 40)

I state that once a pharmaceutical is approved it appears as if it is black boxed because in Canada and the United States, the regulatory organizations rely on pharmaceutical manufacturers to self-report any ongoing pharmaceutical testing and also to report any adverse effects caused by their products. In addition, pharmaceutical companies often promise postmarketing clinical trials as a condition of approval, yet as of 2006, more than 70% of these promised studies have not been started (Avorn, 2007). This implies that pharmaceutical safety is compromised by the apparent failure of pharmaceutical manufacturers to conduct postmarketing studies as well as government regulators who allow such practices to continue (Public Citizen's Health Research Group, 2001). Clearly, we cannot rely on manufacturers to collect, analyze, and report any ongoing research data, as they possess very obvious vested interests.

As mentioned earlier, in the United States the FDA has "very limited resources to conduct post-marketing pharmaceutical safety surveillance" (Miller, 2007). Furthermore, the small percentage of user fees that are permitted to go to postmarket surveillance is insufficient to conduct even one large-scale study on serious pharmaceutical-associated cardiovascular risks associated with a single class of pharmaceuticals (Hennessy & Strom, 2007, p. 1703). Yet, in the United States, as in Canada, the FDA

FIGURE 5. Status of 1,259 commitments for postmarketing studies on pharmaceuticals requested by the FDA, as of September 30, 2006.

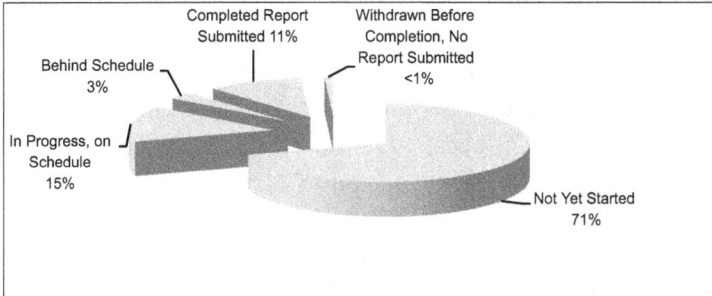

Completed Report
Submitted 11%

Withdrawn Before
Completion, No
Report Submitted
<1%

Behind Schedule
3%

In Progress, on
Schedule
15%

Not Yet Started
71%

Source. Data collected from the U.S. *Federal Register* and cited in Avorn (2007, p. 1697).

is ill-equipped because it does not have the legal authority to compel compliance (Kondro, 2007). As in Canada, the FDA expects the pharmaceutical companies to report adverse effects, and as such, this will require major changes in funding and direction for Health Canada and the FDA if we expect ongoing unbiased pharmaceutical testing postapproval.

Stemming from my analysis of many governmental and academic documents and articles, my findings indicate that while certain pharmaceuticals appear to be black boxed after they are officially approved for sale on the market, they are not always *truly* black boxed, as evidenced by the uncertainties and "loose ends" left unanswered and glossed over prior to approval for both pemoline (as was evidenced by the product's monograph) and tolcapone (as was evidenced by numerous adverse reactions occurring in preapproval clinical trials and highlighted in the product monograph). It appears that what made the networks of actors that included each of the pharmaceuticals in question more or less vulnerable to failure stemmed from this stage of preapproval. As it became apparent to me during the course of my research, the relative strengths on each side of the risk–benefit equation during the approval of each pharmaceutical have major links to whether or not each pharmaceutical will be withdrawn. After all, for both pemoline and tolcapone, a major area of concern during preapproval clinical testing was, indeed, that of hepatic effects. These effects initially concern the liver, yet quickly spread to other areas because, due to the liver's many functions, once the liver is damaged by the pharmaceutical, further negative system-wide adverse effects occur. Not surprisingly, hepatic effects were the main reason for adverse reactions, which led to withdrawal in the cases of both drugs. There were, however, many other organs and systems affected by the adverse effects of both pharmaceuticals, beginning in the preapproval clinical trials. Due to the limitations in preapproval clinical trials, it appears that the more adverse effects in these short trials, the more likely it is that there may possibly exist many and more serious adverse effects in "real life" usage, which will manifest as serious patient illnesses and possibly deaths later on. In effect, the more uncertainty and safety considerations in existence at the preapproval stage of the pharmaceutical's "lifespan," the more vulnerable it is to safety concerns, and as a result, susceptibility to withdrawal later on.

Safer et al. (2001) noted that adverse pharmaceutical reaction reports wherein pemoline was the suspected agent had been sent to the FDA steadily since the pharmaceutical was introduced in 1975. Between 1975 and 1996, 1,296 such reports concerning pemoline were sent directly to the FDA by health professionals or indirectly to the FDA by Abbott Laboratories. Individuals younger than the age of 20 were the focus of 75% of reports with a listed age.[6] The male-to-female ratio was 4 to 1 when gender was reported. Furthermore, there were relatively few serious outcome reports between 1975 and 1980, although six cases of jaundice were reported then. During the period from 1981 to 1985, serious outcome reports were at or near their peak, and they remained generally at that level for the next 10 years (Safer et al., 2001). There were 71 reports of serious outcomes from 1975 through 1996 where pemoline was the suspected agent. Adverse pharmaceutical reaction reports over this period included 24 cases of jaundice and 9 hepatotoxic deaths (Safer et al., 2001).

Although a large number of adverse reaction reports concerning pemoline were received by the FDA over the years, it is important to note that the FDA does not regularly report to the medical community how many adverse reaction reports it has received (Psaty et al., 2004). As a result, the only way for physicians to have been made aware of pemoline's adverse effects was through the scientific literature. Unlike the steady rate of hepatotoxic adverse pharmaceutical reaction reports concerning pemoline that went directly or indirectly to the FDA, however, based on my pemoline database, relatively few reports of serious pemoline toxicity were published in the medical literature.

Between 1975 and 1990, only two letters to the editor reported pemoline hepatotoxicity. Safer et al. (2001) reported on both of these letters: The first in 1984 was of a case of a 10-year-old boy who had abnormal liver function test results after 4 weeks of treatment with pemoline. The liver function test results remained abnormal for 3 weeks after the treatment ceased. A rechallenge later with a low dose of pemoline did not lead to recurrent toxicity (Patterson, 1984, as cited in Safer et al., 2001). Safer et al. also reported on the second letter to the editor in 1989 which "was based on a request by a medical practitioner to the manufacturer for information on two pemoline-related deaths that he had heard about" from another physician (p. 624). The letter described the findings from the manufacturer's files of two deaths attributed to pemoline (Jaffe, 1989, as cited in Safer et al.). Furthermore, "in 1990, four cases of hepatotoxic reactions ascribed to pemoline were published in three brief papers in the gastroenterology literature" (Safer et al., p. 624). In congruence with my database, since 1995 published reports of pemoline hepatotoxicity, liver transplants, and death have increased with more written each year (Safer et al, 2001). In effect, medical literature reports of adverse pharmaceutical reactions associated with pemoline treatment were primarily published in the 1990s, in contrast to the constant flow of adverse pharmaceutical reaction reports to the FDA since 1975 (Safer et al.). The most recent addition of the *Physicians' Desk Reference* makes reference to 13 cases of acute hepatic failure that have been reported to the FDA. Pliszka (1998) noted that these additional cases were not reported anywhere in the scientific literature at the time.

In effect, there was a delay of 1 to 2 decades in the medical community's awareness of the scope of hepatotoxic adverse pharmaceutical reaction reports associated with pemoline use. Liver transplants secondary to pemoline hepatotoxicity were reported in the medical literature in 1995 (one case; Berkovitch et al., 1995, as cited in Safer et al., 2001) and in 1998 (three cases; Adcock et al., 1998, as cited in Safer et al.; Rosh et al., 1998, as cited in Safer et al.). Although 12 cases of jaundice and six deaths ascribed to pemoline in youths were reported to the FDA before 1988, none had been reported in the medical literature during that period (Safer et al., 2001). Safer et al. believed that this delay in awareness of the linkage between pemoline and its associated adverse effects can be ascribed to the following reasons: In the majority of the adverse reactions, liver toxicity occurred 5 or more months after the beginning of treatment with pemoline; of those who did have elevated liver enzymes (a sign of liver damage), the great majority had no physical symptoms; the majority of those who developed jaundice due to pemoline-induced liver damage eventually got better; and "delays in the spontaneous reporting of rare and late-onset adverse pharmaceutical events for certain pharmaceuticals are not uncommon" (p. 626).

In the case of tolcapone, it is true that Health Canada ordered its withdrawal from the market after three patient deaths, but there was evidence of many other adverse effects reported to Health Canada before this, including uncertainties and doubts over the drug's safety during the initial medical review of clinical trials for approval (Tolcapone Product Monograph, 1998). Furthermore, other adverse reaction reports were submitted continuously while the pharmaceutical was in use by the general public. In the current situation, then, once the pharmaceutical is approved, it appears to be black boxed until the risks in its risk–benefit equation are documented to clearly overshadow potential benefits for patients, a new pharmaceutical with a more favorable risk–benefit equation is introduced for the condition, and/or major public interest groups step up, as in Public Citizen's campaign to withdraw pemoline off the American market. From this, it appears that once a certain risk "threshold" is reached behind the closed doors of Health Canada and the FDA, the pharmaceutical is considered for reevaluation or withdrawal, after which the appearance of a "closed" black box falls apart (if it is indeed ordered for withdrawal). Hence, the pharmaceuticals in question, pemoline and tolcapone, serve as examples of the failure of the black box to "hold together" and stay closed which thereby causes each network to fail and be replaced by other networks.

The sociology of translation, an important concept in ANT, expresses how innovations are translated or constructed and transposed from one state to another and how different actors may be co-opted, or enrolled, to support a particular innovation or project within a heterogeneous network of actors (Callon, 1986, as cited in Klecun, 2004, p. 265). Klecun noted that "for a network to succeed or be sustained, such a transformation must become stable (stronger) and even irreversible; however, this stability is often difficult to sustain" (Klecun, p. 265). This is because technologies are not simply marketed and taken up by passive consumers, but rather are shaped by consumers by how they respond to and translate these technologies for their own purposes, often shifting the original reasons for, and methods of, use of such technologies, and in the process creating new or bigger networks (Williams-Jones & Graham, 2003). Latour (1994) wrote that in implementing a new technology, it may be necessary to allow it to drift into unexpected situations because if the technology is going to work, it must be open to change. "Innovations configure the user, defining who may use it and how, but they also modify existing social structures and create new ones" (Williams-Jones & Graham, 2003, p. 277). This was exemplified in the case of pemoline, which was employed off-label (outside the scope of the approved uses of the pharmaceutical) by an estimated 10,000 Americans afflicted with the sleep disorders of narcolepsy and idiopathic hypersomnia, conditions for which it was never intended or tested.

In her novel analysis of methadone from an ANT perspective, Emilie Gomart wrote, "Whether conscious or not, this actant, the patient is key" (2002, p. 118). After all, it is important to remember that "treatments succeed or fail depending on the compliance and personality of the user, not the properties of the substance" alone (Gomart, 2002, p. 118). In the case of pharmaceutical approval and withdrawal, I have stated that one must ask critical questions of reviewers and scientists as they pour over submissions—are they truly unbiased and rational in their decision making? The same can be asked of patients who report on their well-being after testing pharmaceuticals in clinical trials or thereafter. Just as one cannot assume that pharmaceutical manufacturers, reviewers, and prescribing physicians are naturally objective and rational, so, too, one cannot assume this of patients. It is possible that underlying illnesses or beliefs altered how patients reported on their physical ailments while on pemoline or tolcapone. This has been demonstrated regularly in clinical trials under the "placebo effect." The placebo effect occurs when a patient's symptoms are alleviated or exacerbated in some way by the treatment in question due to the individual expecting or believing that it will work. In the cases of pemoline and tolcapone, compliance and reporting of adverse effects could be affected by patient characteristics ranging from severity of the medical condition and willingness to accept adverse effects to the convenience of dosing in the case of pemoline. The latter point was clearly demonstrated by Abbott Laboratories' decision to discontinue sales of pemoline once they had declined to less than US$1 million a year (Knowles, 2005, p. 62). At the time of approval, pemoline was the only ADHD medication available which allowed once-a-day dosing. Due to the development of long-acting formulations of standard stimulant medications, this was no longer a unique characteristic, but rather one which was shared by other medications. Coupled with increasingly prevalent adverse reaction reports and Health Canada's warning that the drug only be considered as a second-line pharmaceutical therapy for ADHD (Keung & Daly, 1998), these factors undoubtedly led to the dissolution of pemoline's appeal to patients and physicians.

Latour wrote that "when a fact is not believed, when an innovation is not taken up, when a theory is put to a completely different use, the model [of ANT] simply says that 'some groups resist'" (1987, p. 135). This point, wherein bureaucrats, physicians, and patients no longer believe in, approve of, or administer a pharmaceutical, constitutes a failure of the black boxing of a subject, resulting in a breakdown, or failure, of the network upon which it relies and which relies on it. This moment exemplifies what Latour described as

> the black box moving in space and becoming durable in time only through the actions of many people; if there is no one to take it up, it stops and falls apart regardless of however many people may have taken it up for however long before. (p. 137)

In short, there is nothing static, stable, or permanent about any one network.

The cases of tolcapone and pemoline also serve to demonstrate that there failed to be any one central actor or ultimate source of power in each network. In each respective case, it may be that either tolcapone or pemoline appeared to be at the center of each network and by extension, hold ultimate power in it. However, if and when each pharmaceutical ceases to be approved, be believed in, prescribed, and administered, or to adequately "work" and be withdrawn from the market, each pharmaceutical will no longer serve as a focal point in the network. In this case, the pharmaceutical's ultimate power can be disputed because researchers, approval boards, physicians, and ultimately patients can be seen as sequentially having ultimate power. Researchers decide how much testing and/ or alterations of the chemical properties will occur, approval boards decide to approve and/or withdraw the pharmaceutical, physicians decided to prescribe it or not, and patients choose to purchase and administer the pharmaceutical or not. Hence, the possession of power in the network is relative to the perspective taken and effectively rests with each member of the network.

5.6. ANALYZING INTERNATIONAL LINKS

> *One of the dilemmas that pharmaceutical companies
> face is making the pharmaceutical [development
> and approval] process more predictable and thereby
> ensuring product development and market share. To
> make the [process] more predictable companies aspire
> to control settings and activities outside the domain of
> industry.*
>
> —Mather (2005, p. 1324)

As mentioned before, pharmaceutical sales approval and withdrawal in the country of manufacture has importance not only for that particular country, but also for licensing decisions in other countries, although not directly (Abraham & Lawton Smith, 2003). One could surmise that pharmaceutical approval and withdrawal is monitored and harmonized internationally, although this, in fact, has not been the case, resulting in my exploration into why such large discrepancies in time and mode of action exist between the two federal departments in commanding market withdrawals of the same pharmaceuticals.

The International Conference on Harmonization of Technical Requirements for Registration of Pharmaceuticals for Human Use (ICH) attempted to standardize pharmaceutical regulation internationally beginning in the late 1980s. Such standardization in member countries undoubtedly served as a means of strengthening the network of manufacturers applying for pharmaceutical approval by creating a centrality of power and knowledge in specific places at their disposal. With one set of guidelines and requirements and one source for this (much-reduced) required information, it appears highly likely that the actors who benefit most from the ICH are indeed the manufacturers. Although more streamlined requirements internationally could be advantageous to organizations scrutinizing pharmaceuticals for approval, since a very limited number of countries are directly involved, this appears to be secondary in purpose. Nonetheless, the standardized regulations put into effect by the ICH continue to be in effect today with supporters located worldwide as well as in powerful organizations such as the World Health Organization (WHO; Abraham & Lawton Smith, 2003).

The predicament with the ICH is the fact that its key participants are the three pharmaceutical industry associations and the three government pharmaceutical regulatory agencies of the European Union, Japan, and the United States—the three largest pharmaceutical markets in the world (Nakajima, 1996). Together, these six cosponsors form the core of the ICH network of pharmaceutical industry and government scientists, who have, in effect, become a transnational power in setting the regulatory standards on the safety, quality, and efficacy of new prescription medicines. As a result, the standards for new pharmaceutical approval developed by the ICH have been invariably adopted by the government regulatory agencies of the European Union, Japan, and the United States throughout the 1990s (Abraham & Lawton Smith, 2003). The steering committee of the ICH comprises two representatives with voting rights from each of the six cosponsors. The International Federation of Pharmaceutical Manufacturers and Associations (IFPMA) provides the secretariat for the steering committee, who selects the "technical" topics for regulatory harmonization and appoints "expert working groups" of professional scientists. The membership of these groups is not fixed, but rather each of the six cosponsors can nominate a leader and deputy leader for each group, and most members are scientists from either the industry or government regulatory agencies (D'Arcy & Harron, 1998, as cited in Abraham & Lawton Smith, 2003).

Before the ICH, most of the 17 regulatory agencies in the European Union, Japan, and the United States required expedited reporting (i.e., within a matter of days) of serious, nonserious, or both adverse pharmaceutical reactions, even if they were expected with the new pharmaceutical (Garutti, 1994). However, opting for a more lenient directive, the ICH recommended that expedited reporting to regulators "is not generally appropriate for expected, unrelated, or non-serious cases" (Gordon, 1994, as cited in Abraham, 2002b, p. 1500). The ICH also adopted a low standard when considering the carcinogenic risk to patients in clinical trials. Even though Japanese and American regulators require that clinical trial data must be collected for 12 months before a pharmaceutical is eligible to receive marketing approval, and the FDA requires the submission of carcinogenicity testing for pharmaceuticals that will be administered to trial patients for more than 3 months, the ICH recommended that no carcinogenicity testing be completed on compounds which will be administered to patients in clinical trials for less than 6 months (Abraham, 2002b; International Conference on Harmonization, 1995).

> Similarly, the regulatory agencies agreed to reduce the minimum duration of patients' treatment in clinical trials from 12 to 6 months in initial marketing applications, despite research made available to them showing that about a quarter of serious [adverse drug reactions] that happened in clinical trials of 1 year duration arose after 6 months. (Abraham, 2002b, p. 1500)

In effect, it appears that the ICH, rather than serving as a first step towards an objective international regulatory synchronization, has instead become a means of streamlining burdensome regulatory requirements for pharmaceutical manufacturers.

There is no doubt that many in the transnational pharmaceutical industry regard the ICH as the first step towards global harmonization of regulatory standards and the production of a "global registration dossier," which would contain all of the types of data required for new pharmaceutical approval in any country in the world (Abraham & Lawton Smith, 2003, p. 85). As a senior official at the pharmaceutical manufacturer Glaxo Wellcome commented,

> We found these different tests and differences in regulations delayed our time to get to market. There was a ground swell from industry that for certain safety testing, these differences were unnecessary. *The ICH was developed to reduce redundant testing* [italics added]. The driver initially was to reduce the number of animals in safety testing. It then expanded to cover quality, safety and efficacy. The industry supports it because in order to cut costs what we want to do is to have one global pharmaceutical development package covering quality, safety and efficacy that can be applicable to all regulatory applications in the three regions. We hope and anticipate that the same package will also be acceptable in the other 141 countries of the WHO. (Abraham & Lawton Smith, 2003, p. 84)

Based on my findings, it is important to note that Health Canada and the FDA are not "connected" in any direct fashion, nor do they share pharmaceutical information of any kind, at least not officially. Hence, if one country conducts research, testing, and decision making on a particular substance, there is no requirement that the other should be consulted, enlightened, or that it must follow in its footsteps regarding regulation. The ICH is a project that attempted to streamline and standardize pharmaceutical regulation internationally, most directly in Europe, Japan, and the United States. Canadian regulatory authorities are not involved as key members in the ICS; however, they have already adopted some scientific standards put forth by the key members (Health Canada, 1999). Membership in the ICH does not, however, require any country to share its research with others or for others to update it on their research. Furthermore, it appears that the ICH's main goals affected the simplification of approval procedures for pharmaceutical manufacturers but not regulators or those dealing with postapproval research or withdrawal. All of this information raises the question of how changes in regulation and approval requirements affect the likelihood of pharmaceutical withdrawal later on. After all, more permissive regulations, as the ICH ones appear to be, undoubtedly allow for pharmaceuticals with greater potential for compromising patient safety to be approved and employed by the public.

5.7. ANALYZING DIFFERENCES BETWEEN CANADA AND THE UNITED STATES

The insight of Bodewitz, Buurma, and de Vries (1987, p. 244, as cited in Abraham & Davis, 2007, p. 410) that the interests and expectations of different groups become linked in the institutional and professional networks of pharmaceutical regulation is a helpful starting point in understanding why there were such contrasting Canadian and American regulatory expectations. How different was the Canadian pemoline approval and withdrawal process from the American? How different was the Canadian tolcapone approval and withdrawal process from the American? One might expect that the Canadian and American treatments of the pharmaceuticals in question converged to reveal, even vaguely, an identical underlying pharmaceutical compound in terms of the final outcomes imposed. Strikingly, however, it is just at this point that the variations and multiplicities of performances of both pharmaceuticals are most numerous.

In analyzing documents submitted to both Health Canada and the FDA in order to gain approval for both pharmaceuticals, I discovered that there is very little, if any difference, between data submitted by each manufacturer to each reviewing body. The same documentation of clinical trials and results, environmental assessments, statistical reviews, and pharmacological details were submitted. In effect, both pharmaceuticals were approved in both countries based on the same data and with little difference in reviewers' notes and apprehensions. The difference between the two countries in question, rather, appears to be varying approval and withdrawal thresholds. From my research, it appears that the key is varying criteria—there are no set rules or guidelines steering the withdrawal of a previously approved pharmaceutical in either country. I believe that it is precisely this variation in criteria, views, perspectives, and ways of measuring terms in the risk–benefit equation that allows each country's regulatory organization to proceed as it feels is necessary with each case submitted for approval and also for withdrawal. Armed with the power to assess each pharmaceutical uniquely from others, regulators may decide for or against approval or withdrawal, possibly swayed by factors such as patient groups, advisory committees and their individual members' partialities, and lobbyists. In effect, each pharmaceutical is seen differently and treated differently in each country. As a result, how can one expect synchronicity between Canada and the United States when they do not have synchronicity amongst themselves regarding one pharmaceutical as compared to another?

From my analysis of reviewer's documents, I have also discovered that much of the approval or withdrawal-related decision making has to do with the existence and effectiveness of other approved pharmaceuticals for the medical condition in question (as was the case for pemoline in both Canada and the United States) or the lack of (as was the case for tolcapone). Judging from the cases of pemoline and tolcapone then, patient deaths only seem to matter if something safer exists. It appears that something is always better than nothing regarding pharmaceutical treatments for specific conditions. This point appears to have been a key aspect influencing the safety threshold of both pemoline and tolcapone.

In the case of pemoline, other efficacious, yet less harmful (or so it is thought) long-acting pharmaceuticals were available in Canada and the United States beginning in 2001 with Concerta, followed by Dexedrine, Adderall XR, and Ritalin-SR (the once-a-day dose of Ritalin)—all vital nonhuman actors, which in effect sounded the death knoll for its popularity. Health Canada decided to actively withdraw pemoline for this reason along with the fact that specific evidence supporting its safety was not provided by the manufacturer. In its *Canadian Adverse Drug Reaction Newsletter* from January of 2000, Health Canada defended its decision based on the following considerations:

> Despite explicit warnings in the product monograph and labelling information regarding the risk of severe liver damage, worldwide case reports of liver failure necessitating transplantation or resulting in death continued; there is no evidence that liver damage caused by the pharmaceutical is predictable or reversible; other, safer treatment alternatives are available; and a satisfactory response to the Therapeutic Product Programme's request for specific evidence to support the safety of the pharmaceutical's continued use was not provided by the manufacturer. (Health Canada, 2000, p. 3)

The FDA did not actively withdraw the pharmaceutical, but by the end of 2005, the manufacturer had discontinued it due to low sales volumes. The reality of low sales likely affected Abbott Laboratories' decision to forego investment into Health Canada's required "evidence" for the pharmaceutical since it is very likely that the manufacturer was aware of decreasing sales in Canada as in the United States, and thus expected to discontinue sales in Canada in the near future had the pharmaceutical not been withdrawn by the regulatory authorities first. Meanwhile, throughout the time period in question, it appears that the FDA was simply too occupied or too underfunded to undergo an entire withdrawal review process for a pharmaceutical which it considered relatively unused and unimportant. One may ask whether the FDA would withdraw a more widely used drug with the same safety profile. One cannot answer for certain, although, as Hennessy and Strom (2007) noted, under the current arrangement under the PDUFA agreement in the United States, the risks of pharmaceuticals already on the market receive little attention, and the FDA has very limited resources to conduct postmarketing pharmaceutical safety surveillance with only 5% of user fees permitted to go to postmarketing surveillance.

Regarding tolcapone, Health Canada also withdrew the pharmaceutical based on its checkered safety history, wherein serious adverse reactions began in clinical trials and continued throughout the patient population upon approval, as well as the upcoming approval of other, less harmful pharmaceuticals in the same class. This latter point appears to be central as to why tolcapone was approved for use in Canada in the first place. At the time, in 1997, there was no other therapeutic product available in Canada which could be prescribed to Parkinson's disease patients in order to prolong the treatment effects of their primary medication, levodopa. Even so, tolcapone was still indicated as a second-line pharmaceutical for those who were "not responding satisfactorily to or [were] not appropriate candidates for other adjunctive therapies" (Tolcapone Product Monograph, 1998, p. 3). Orion, a Finnish company, was in the process of receiving approval for entacapone which would function identically to tolcapone, but which only gained Health Canada's approval in May of 2001. Patients on entacapone, however, although also experiencing adverse reactions such as dyskinesia and nausea, did not suffer from diarrhea and most importantly, hepatic effects were not observed (Kieburtz & Hubble, 2000).

It appears that tolcapone was approved hastily in order to prevent delays in a specific subset of patients' access to an important new class of pharmaceuticals any longer than necessary. With subsequent serious adverse effects clearly caused by tolcapone, Health Canada decided to withdraw the pharmaceutical nonetheless, verifying that it had made a mistake in approving a medication which simply had more risks than benefits, as compared to more benefits than risks as had been expected. The FDA, in contrast, chose to continue the approval of tolcapone, albeit with stringent product warnings, stating that with proper medical supervision, the product had merit also for those "not responding satisfactorily to or [who were] not appropriate candidates for other adjunctive therapies" (Tolcapone Product Monograph, 1998, p. 3). On the FDA Web site, tolcapone is still referred to as the sole therapeutic treatment for adjunct treatment with levodopa for Parkinson's disease with "no therapeutic equivalents" (Food and Drug Administration—Center for Drug Evaluation and Research, 2008, p. 1), although entacapone (another COMT inhibitor in the same class of pharmaceuticals) received approval there in October of 1999. Tolcapone may be seen as having "no therapeutic equivalents" because it is has been proven to be slightly more effective than entacapone at decreasing "off times" in Parkinson's patients (Kieburtz & Hubble, 2000), although its risks, particularly those related to the liver, likely outweigh the benefits for most physicians and patients.

In both pharmaceutical cases profiled, Health Canada appears to have been more stringent regarding the withdrawal of harmful pharmaceuticals off the market with the FDA lagging behind by first issuing warning letters and black box warnings prior to actually withdrawing the pharmaceuticals. This does not appear to be a significant pattern when all pharmaceutical withdrawals between the two countries were compared from 1963 to 2004 (Rawson & Kaitin, 2003). In their study, Rawson and Kaitin compared new pharmaceutical approval times in Canada and the United States over a 10-year period and related them to each country's withdrawals. They found that new pharmaceutical approval times were significantly longer in Canada than in the United States, but due to this, Canada avoided potential dangers because its longer approval times provided an opportunity to observe actual market experience in other countries. Hence, when serious safety problems were identified in a timely manner after American approval, the pharmaceuticals were not subsequently approved in Canada. However, the trade-off is that new products, including those for conditions for which current therapy has limited efficacy, take significantly longer to be approved in Canada and, hence, to be available to Canadians. It is interesting to note, however, that there is poor concordance between pharmaceuticals that receive priority review in Canada and those that undergo accelerated review in the United States (Rawson, 2005, as cited in Marra et al., 2006). Clearly, this is a key issue which remains unexplained and to which my book helps to provide an answer.

After all, it is more than likely that the same factors which effectuated such diversity in approval and withdrawal decisions regarding pemoline and tolcapone are at work regarding decisions about other pharmaceuticals, including those undergoing expedited review. This again refers back to the usage of varying criteria, views, and perspectives by Canadian and American authorities during pharmaceutical review, which essentially results in different risk–benefit equations on both sides of the border. As a result, the pharmaceutical being scrutinized for approval or withdrawal changes depending on which country it is being reviewed in.

There has been discussion in the literature regarding the length of time for approval of pharmaceuticals in Canada, which currently rests at about 300 days for a new pharmaceutical submission (Kelly et al., 2007). Historically, Canada has had pharmaceutical approval times that are similar to those in Australia, but longer than those reported for the United Kingdom and the United States (Lexchin, 2006b; Rawson & Kaitin, 2003). However, as mentioned previously, Rawson and Kaitin (2003) demonstrated that although pharmaceutical approval times in Canada are longer than in the United States[7], the proportion of new pharmaceuticals approved in Canada but later discontinued for safety reasons was lower in the Canadian market (2.0%) as compared with the United States (3.6%) in a 10-year period from 1992 to 2001, suggesting that the Canadian approval process is more stringent.

5.8. IMPLICATIONS FOR CURRENT REGULATORY THINKING

Although I am aware that in general ANT tends to abstain from moral and political viewpoints and commentary, I believe that it is nonetheless of utmost importance to provide the reader of this book a series of thoughts and practical policy implications which can be taken away and acted upon in order to improve portions of our political and medical systems. It is my hope that we can control and prevent some of the negative issues and actors influencing our pharmaceutical and medical care discussed within this book. After all, it is of utmost importance to be able to "grab onto something" tangible with practical implications for change; change which many individuals and authors state is much needed. In the end, I wrote this book with the intention that it would serve as a jolt to those who read it—there is no question that the matters within it are serious. I did not want to do this by fear-mongering or dramatization, but rather by stating the facts and allowing the reader to make their own conclusions. As a result, I really do hope that each reader can take what he or she feels is most important from my findings and act on them accordingly. What follows is an overview of what is being done and can be done in Canada in order to improve "the system."

In the wake of the Vioxx "fiasco," Health Canada and other regulatory agencies worldwide are reexamining how they approve and monitor pharmaceuticals under the term of a "progressive licensing framework" (Health Canada, 2007; Hébert, 2007). "Health Canada states that its version of progressive licensing includes the development of an increasingly patient-centered focus," the improved gathering and synthesis of evidence on pharmaceuticals beginning at the development stage, as well as the improvement of postmarketing pharmaceutical safety surveillance (Hébert, 2007, p. 1801). As a result, the agency is now gathering information and forming drafts for consultation (Yeates, Lee, & Maher, 2007).

Based on existing literature, the progressive licensing framework appears to include forthcoming changes to both legislation and regulations in order to enhance both the steps necessary for pharmaceutical approval and for postmarketing surveillance (Health Canada, 2007; Hébert, 2007; Yeates et al., 2007). As Hébert (2007) noted, these changes may result in the threshold for approval of new pharmaceuticals being lower in exchange for more stringent rules pertaining to the continuous evaluation of pharmaceuticals after they are approved. Although such changes can provide quicker access to new treatments, they could also mean that hazardous ones are available for use before they are tested sufficiently, as was the case with both pemoline and tolcapone.

In congruence with other authors, I believe that in order to have significant and consequential reform, however, Health Canada must be immune to the influence of the pharmaceutical industry (Avorn, 2007; Hébert, 2007; Ross, 2007). Otherwise, a situation analogous to the ICH and its apparently self-serving regulations could result. One proposed theory to confer better immunity to Health Canada from the financial and ideological interests of the pharmaceutical industry has been to invite the Canadian Academies of Science (the Canadian version of the American National Academy of Sciences, which oversees the IOM) or the Canadian Academy of Health Sciences (Canada's version of the American IOM) to compose a panel advising parliament, with minimal representation from the pharmaceutical industry (Hébert, 2007). Representatives should be appointed from major Canadian stakeholder groups, including the public, physicians, and regulators, in order to better balance the public's needs with what regulators do. Furthermore, representatives from successful foreign regulatory agencies could lend ideas and standards which have worked in order countries and which could work in Canada. This, too, would serve to better align and harmonize Canada's regulatory standards with international ones, owing to the recognition "that the development and monitoring of drugs is now occurring on a global scale" (Yeates et al., 2007, p. 1845). All of these perspectives have much to add to the "two-note symphony of industry and Health Canada" (Hébert, 2007, p. 1801).

The present pharmaceutical regulatory systems in Canada, the United States, and around the world are insufficiently resilient in their relations with the pharmaceutical industry because they "prevent proper accountability, are highly vulnerable to industrial outsourcing, and permit industry scientists to maintain extensive conflicts of interest while providing their expert advice" to governmental organizations (Abraham, 2002b, p. 1501). A regulatory system which can produce and provide pharmaceutical testing and jurisdiction over pharmaceutical manufacturers solely in the interests of the public is needed. Second, as has been proposed previously (Abraham, 2002b), regulatory agencies should identify key safety tests for each new pharmaceutical application, as well as those necessary for adequate postmarketing surveillance, which their own scientists could then undertake. The cost of these studies could be borne by the companies, but the regulatory agencies would control, own, and publish the data (Abraham, 2002b). This data could then be shared with other regulatory agencies, serving to bring into effect interagency harmonization. In addition to developing technical expertise in pharmaceutical testing within regulatory organizations, this would aid in making regulatory agencies less dependent on recruitment from industry, and such cooperation would undoubtedly assist in bringing about interagency synchronization (Abraham, 2002b). As has been illustrated, there are large disparities between Canadian and American pharmaceutical regulatory policy, in both approval and withdrawal of pharmaceuticals. What is needed is a cooperative international framework wherein pharmaceutical regulatory agencies examine and exchange information routinely, resulting in an environmental conducive to teamwork and analogous guidelines. As Hébert noted, "such harmonization may yield uniform and widely accepted high standards, avoid needless duplication of work, increase trust, and, perhaps eventually, lead to synergistic areas of expertise in either clinical content or research methods" (2007, p. 1801). Clearly, the ICH was arranged to do this but has failed miserably, with no comprehensive or truly valuable regulations currently being adhered to internationally as a result of the meeting of its members.

Currently, premarket approval only requires two Phase 3 trials in highly selective patients (Hébert, 2007). These yield little data in small numbers of "perfect" patients. As part of the improvement to the approval process, the progressive licensing framework panel could insist that new pharmaceuticals undergo large trials with "realistic" patient populations consisting of those who would actually take the pharmaceutical in question. These reviews could "yield meaningful results," as demonstrated recently by the cardiac-risk warning attached by the FDA to rosiglitazone (Avandia®), a diabetes drug (Hébert, 2007, p. 1801; Nissen & Wolski, 2007). The original approval of rosiglitazone was based on the ability of the drug to reduce blood glucose and hemoglobin levels. However, the manufacturer's studies did not adequately determine the effects of the pharmaceutical on associated complications of diabetes, including cardiovascular morbidity and mortality. As Nissen and Wolski noted however, "[T]he effect of any antidiabetic therapy on cardiovascular outcomes is particularly important, because more than 65% of deaths in patients with diabetes are from cardiovascular causes" (p. 2458). The authors found that rosiglitazone was, in fact, associated with a significant increase in the risk of myocardial infarction (heart attack) and with an increase in the risk of death from cardiovascular causes. In their discussion, they noted that

> the FDA considers demonstration of a sustained reduction in blood glucose levels with an acceptable safety profile adequate for approval of antidiabetic agents. However, the ultimate value of antidiabetic therapy is the reduction of the complications of diabetes, not [solely] improvement in a laboratory measure of glycemic control. After the apparent increase in adverse cardiovascular outcomes with rosiglitazone, the use of blood glucose measurements as a surrogate end point in regulatory approval must be carefully re-examined. (p. 2469)

In addition to subjecting new pharmaceuticals to large pragmatic trials with realistic patient subsets, it would be wise to examine the current pharmaceutical regulatory system in order to determine whether, for example, we may be better served by increased separation between the pharmaceutical approval and postmarket surveillance functions and by increased powers (and funding) for appropriate pharmaceutical monitoring. Next, national governments should reassert more responsibility for funding regulatory review so that appropriate agencies do not have to depend on industry fees to do their work. Finally, expert advisers to regulatory agencies should be required to suspend all conflicts of interest during their time in office.

It is true that "the worldwide withdrawal of Vioxx marked the end of an era of relative consumer innocence" (Hébert, 2007, p. 1801). This high-exposure withdrawal demonstrated unequivocally that, unlike other consumer "goods," pharmaceutical products cannot be driven by profit (Hébert, p. 1801). Rather, the goal must be a transparent, patient-centered regulatory system that ensures pharmaceuticals are safe and efficacious before and after their release. Pharmaceutical manufacturers must provide access to all information on pharmaceutical safety in a timely and usable fashion, perhaps by posting major results in public trial registries (Laine et al., 2007).

There must be greater cooperation between all levels of government in each country and between the governments of each country so that all necessary information can be accessed by researchers and interested parties prior to major adverse reactions actually reaching the public.

ENDNOTES

1. Mather also saw actors in the way that Latour described them, namely, that actors can be both human and nonhuman entities. He noted, however, that he used the term in "a more dated way, conforming to the dramaturgical model wherein all the world is a stage and we all [including non-human actors] have roles..." (C. M. Mather, personal communication, March 10, 2008).

2. In 2004 Celebrex sales comprised 75%, or US$3.3 billion, of pain reliever sales. In December of that same year during the week when news of its cardiovascular risk became public, Celebrex claimed 44% of prescription painkiller sales in the retail market with revenues of US$44 million. By February 11 of 2005, Celebrex's share fell to 23% with sales of US$24 million (Kaledin, 2005).

3. The acne drug Accutane (isotretinoin) was introduced in 1983 and became one of the most effective prescription drugs available for acne. With time, it became apparent that Accutane is highly teratogenic: It can cause severe birth defects when taken during pregnancy. About one quarter of babies born who have been exposed to Accutane during gestation have major congenital deformities. Those babies born without major malformations frequently develop severe learning disabilities later on. Almost half of all "Accutane babies" do not survive pregnancy: 40% are spontaneously miscarried. This combination of unique and powerful efficacy coupled with serious risk has posed a serious challenge for the FDA over the past 20 years (Honein, Paulozzi and Erickson, 2001).

4. Direct-to-consumer advertisements were allowed by U.S. law beginning in September of 1985, provided that product labeling information was presented with the advertisement. In Canada, limited direct-to-consumer advertising is currently permitted (Morgan, 2007).

5. Dyskinesia refers to involuntary movements. In the context of Parkinson's disease, dyskinesias are often the result of chronic

levodopa therapy. These motor fluctuations occur in more than half of Parkinson's disease patients after 5 to 10 years of levodopa therapy, with the percentage of affected patients increasing over time (Obeso et al., 2000).

6. Out of a total of 951 individuals, there were 716 youths.

7. An average of 317 days in the Canadian system, as compared with 232 days in the U.S. system (Lexchin, 2004).

CHAPTER 6

CONCLUSION

6.1. THE LIMITATIONS OF ACTOR NETWORK THEORY (ANT)

As with any theoretical approach, one can expect some shortcomings when working with ANT. These, of course, stem directly from the directives and rules of employing ANT in the first place. For one, ANT rejects any preconceived distinction between technology and society, instead "proposing that both should be studied in the same way and through the same (or interchangeable) language and metaphors" (Kaplan, 2004, p. 265). As was described in chapter 1, in ANT terms, innovations are developed and adopted (or not) through the building of networks of alliances between human and nonhuman actors (Monteiro, 2000, as cited in Kaplan, 2004). Hence, a major criticism of ANT is directed towards this radical symmetry between human and nonhuman actors, most often because humans are seen to have "morality" wherein machines and corporations do not (Lee & Brown, 1994; Murdoch, 2001; Pickering, 1992; Williams-Jones & Graham, 2003). According to Williams-Jones and Graham (2003), however,

> the purpose of treating humans and non-humans symmetrically is in order to aid in a detailed description of the all-important network, and as such, ANT does not imply or require that all entities be treated as identical for all purposes, nor that the various relations between actors be egalitarian. (p. 278)

Rather, what matters is the "doing" and actions of both humans and nonhumans (therefore *actor network theory*) and the resulting worknets created by their synergistic existence. As was mentioned in chapter 1, actors, whether human or not, do things, and these actions must be responded to. A nonresponse is still classified as a response because a thought process is initiated in the nonresponder.

In a related fashion, ANT's method of analyzing the development of technology has also been criticized for its emphasis on a value neutrality (Kaplan et al., 2004; Walsham, 1997). In their examination of these criticisms, Williams-Jones and Graham (2003) wrote that

> ANT's focus on empirical case studies that provide a rich description of networks has been accused of ignoring the larger social and political context, and thereby undermining the possibility of effective social, ethical and political critique. In this view, ANT perpetuates a functionalist, problem-solving description of networks that can result in collusion with dominant ideologies, such as industry, government or patriarchy (Fuller, 2000; Star, 1991). (p. 278)

Furthermore, Klecun (2004, p. 266) stated that "due to its symmetrical treatment of humans and nonhumans and the definition of action as distributed through different entities (human and nonhuman) in socio-technical assemblies, ANT in particular is open to a charge of diluting intentionality, responsibility and accountability (Latour, 1987; Stalder, 2000)." In addition, "although ANT rejects a priori assignment of motives of actors, it can be argued that implicitly it presumes that actors are rational and goal-oriented" (Klecun, 2004, p. 266).

ANT's main focus was never to provide social or political commentary, but rather to outline and describe the networks from which readers were free to synthesize their own conclusions. As a result, the social scientist is expected to remain value neutral and objective. This does not mean that ANT refuses to accept actors as possessing motives or assumptions, but rather believes that such characteristics must only be exposed during examination of the actors and their actions during the study itself. After all, translation states that each actor, whether composed of an individual or an assembly, is assumed to possess individual interests. In ANT, a network's stability is seen as resulting from this continual translation of interests between actors. Policies, behaviors, motivations, and goals are seen as being translated from one actor to another, and actors are themselves translated and changed in their interactions with others (Callon, 1986). One could argue that having awareness of suspicions or suppositions prior to studying certain actors causes one to focus on specific actions and potential conflicts rather than be completely open minded to the emergence of new or unexpected ones. This is why one must forge ahead doing ANT research with no preconceived ideas about actors or their interests, yet be open to them should they arise.

With the aforementioned points in mind, I nonetheless agree that employing ANT's proposed research method involving the elimination (in an ideal situation) of preconceived ideas and assumptions about actors as well as which actors are involved in a particular network may lead a researcher to overlook or exclude certain actors which do not become readily observable through the research. Perhaps Klecun's (2004) following assertion serves as the most useful in addressing this dilemma:

> An empirical program for critically led research would aim to question the status quo through detailed studies of how things come to be, for which following the actors would be an excellent start, and *also* be sensitive to a priori constructs. Such constructs should not be taken for granted or seen as natural and enduring, but instead act as sensitizers. Empirical study should concentrate on local, situated actions and relationships and see them as historically situated. (p. 270, italics in original)

In this book, I tried to approach actors and networks without preconceived notions of who would be involved or how. Rather, I decided to begin by researching each of the two pharmaceuticals by first examining their histories in detail from preclinical trials onwards, with key additional actors being identified along the way. Further research then went into each actor who had been identified, while I still consciously strove to maintain sensitivity to further actors being discovered. For obvious reasons, I knew from prior research that certain actors, such as pharmaceutical manufacturers and marketing practices, would be linked and likely involved in both networks. Once a significant number of actors were identified in each network, an examination of their linkages and sources of interest in the network was undertaken. Each actor and network was seen as value neutral until proven otherwise. For example, when the pharmaceutical industry in the United States as a whole (Pharmaceutical Research and Manufacturers of America [PhRMA]) was recognized as an actor, it was not ascribed any self-serving characteristics or values until evidence showed otherwise, such as its role in the Prescription Pharmaceutical User Fee Act. Similarly, in order to better understand the review process conducted by the Food and Drug Administration (FDA), I concentrated on local, situated actions and relationships such as the steps involved in reviewing pemoline for withdrawal, yet also recognized that they were historically situated in that they were based on the existence of other newer and safer medications being available for the same condition.

Another criticism of ANT has been its unique view of the micro-macro relationship, in that it believes in a "uniform framework regardless of the unit of analysis" and, as such, "it refuses to distinguish [before the research is actually done] between small and large networks (Callon & Latour, 1981; Monteiro, 2000)" (Klecun, 2004, p. 268). According to Klecun (2004),

> ANT suggests that it is the actors that establish (interpret and make real) the macro trends, and thus we should not create an artificial distinction between the local and the global but that we can extend a study to ever-wider actor-networks. (p. 268)

This approach has been criticized for its circularity. For example, Monteiro (2000, as cited in Klecun, 2004) argued that Latour reduced the terms *society* and *nature* to local actions. Furthermore, Klecun (2004) argued that

> starting with actors involved with an innovation, and not referring to the traditional categories of social theory,

> such as class, culture and the state, means we might not
> be aware of or even concerned about actors (or potential
> actors) who are missing. (p. 268)

As a result, one may not be able to explain why certain actors may have been excluded or marginalized after the fact of the analysis.

It is important to add flesh and rebuttals to these points. My view is that when done correctly, empirical studies employing ANT trace out networks, or relevant parts thereof, in effect linking the micro and macro elements in order to form a "big picture" view of the actors in question and how they are joined and belong together. One can always focus in on a more micro or macro scale of these elements depending on an individual's specific field of study. As was illustrated by figure 1, "the process of identifying the local in the global and vice versa and thus spanning local and global (without making preconceived distinctions) involves boxing or collapsing an entire actor-network into a single actor" (Monteiro, 2000, as cited in Kaplan, 2004, p. 269). Done repeatedly, this results in the network in question coming into focus for study. In this book, this was done by beginning with a single actor, either pemoline or tolcapone, and "opening up" and examining the entire actor network which was black boxed into comprising each pharmaceutical. Hence, stating that one is examining tolcapone, for example, involves identifying the many actors who contributed and continually contribute to the existence of a black box, or node, of tolcapone, including those who were a part of the black box (such as Health Canada in its approval of tolcapone) but who no longer contribute to it.

As can be seen from the aforementioned criticisms and arguments, ANT is not only a theory but also a research method and has the potential to address some of the problems facing the sociologist studying the development of technological advancements, such as those found in the pharmaceutical industry in the case of this book. As a result, ANT develops the necessary concepts and vocabulary in order to assist a researcher in investigating, for example, how networks are formed and how actors are enrolled during early stages of decision-making activities regarding a new pharmaceutical and during its implementation and subsequent use (or nonuse) for treatment (Klecun, 2004, p. 269). ANT also brings to the forefront an original method of viewing and studying human and technological assemblies, which in today's world, exist synergistically and interdependently in almost all fields comprising almost all aspects of daily life. This having been said, it is also up to the researcher to seek and employ the most appropriate aspects of ANT for his or her respective study, all the while addressing its potential shortcomings.

6.2. EXAMINING THE LIMITATIONS OF MY RESEARCH

A key principle of ANT is that from one moment, place, machine, or treatment to the next, a slightly varied version of the object in question is discussed, measured, observed, and treated, depending on the history, interests, and profession of the actor (Mol, 2002). As Mol (p. 5) wrote, "The body, the patient, the disease, the doctor, the technician, the technology; all of these are more than one, more than singular." These multiple views do not, however, imply fragmentation, but rather a multiplicity of the object(s) being studied. Hence, it is undeniable that the same research topic could have been approached, examined, and treated differently depending on which actors were chosen to be of most importance to analyze. The choice regarding which actors are brought to the forefront and which are kept behind, as well as which facets of each are studied, undoubtedly varies depending on the researcher's interests and beliefs. One could see this variability as a shortcoming of this book. Perhaps certain actors are seen as crucial for examination by some readers, yet were not (adequately) examined. Nonetheless, it would be nearly impossible to research, analyze, and examine all actors involved in the specific networks of both pemoline and tolcapone, if only due to time restrictions. In addition, my analysis stems largely from the point of view of a sociological researcher with a biological background, yet of course there are infinite positions from which to see these treatments depending on the researcher's history and interests. In addition, one can see each condition and/or pharmaceutical by focusing in on specific perspectives or nodes in each network, such as patients or physicians rather than the regulatory authorities as I have done.

One could also focus more specifically on the histories of creation of each pharmaceutical by interviewing and researching more directly those involved in the trials and tribulations of the actual synthesis of these pharmaceuticals, or others of interest for that matter. After all, a basic tenant of ANT is that technical and normative values are built into the technology and its supporting documents, marketing, and so forth. As a result, it can be said that human makers can be seen in machines and implements, as well as their work—both disguised under the guise of technology (Latour, 1999). In short, those creating the pharmaceuticals have an important say in their being. Hence, it would be beneficial to understand and examine more about the actual creation of these pharmaceuticals and their "absent makers" (Latour, 1994, p. 40), although such information would be extremely difficult or impossible to obtain from manufacturers, who would most certainly state "privacy concerns" as a reason for withholding it. As mentioned previously, this happened to me during my research, in which case Health Canada was willing to send me more information on pemoline's approval, yet due to privacy concerns cited by the manufacturer, these documents could not be delivered to me. Furthermore, for pharmaceuticals such as pemoline, which were developed and tested decades ago, it is likely that any possible controversies and issues with the chemical compounds at their preliminary research stage have been lost and/or forgotten. What were some of the issues, concerns, and arguments that scientists and those working with the pharmaceuticals had? This is one aspect of the pharmaceuticals' histories which I could not focus on because I did not have access to the necessary information.

Singleton and Michael (1993) wrote that in employing ANT for research, one must recognize and remember that individual actors will change over time, across social and political contexts, and in their relations with other actors. The research which serves as the foundation for this book began in late 2006, and by mid-2008, the situations and relations between the actors in question had likely already changed. Nonetheless, one has to stop data collection at one point and then begin writing and analyzing it. This, however, points to future routes regarding work remaining to be done in this field of research. For one, in synthesizing my research question, I decided to focus primarily on the withdrawal of pharmaceuticals, through which it became clear to me that withdrawal is so closely linked to, and dependent upon, approval. Seeing that the approval processes of both Health Canada and the FDA appear to vary considerably with each pharmaceutical submitted, further juxtaposition and examination of these and other countries' approval and/or withdrawal guidelines and processes is indicated. Apart from comparisons between the United States and United Kingdom (Rawson & Kaitin, 2003), this field is relatively unexplored and, as such, infinite possibilities abound. Similarly, other, newer pharmaceuticals and their differing treatment by both Health Canada and the FDA warrant examination. Furthermore, the gap between withdrawal times in both Canada and the United States appears to be narrowing, with more recent withdrawals occurring within a time span of 5 to 6 years as compared to an all-time variation of 14 years in the 1970s (Rawson & Kaitin; Department of Health and Human Services, 1998b). This, undoubtedly, is a direction that I would like to take with future research stemming from this book.

The comparison of both countries' pharmaceutical-related policies in this book uncovered a lack of unifying regulations and requirements when pharmaceuticals are considered for approval or withdrawal. What remains to be answered is whether or not the status quo has always been this way or when and why it has been altered. Were policies more or less stringent beforehand and, if so, why? Is the current situation in the best interests of the general public or other interested parties? In a related vein, my experience in not being able to obtain documentation for this book has led me to question the difference in how both countries' pharmaceutical control agencies respond to consumer requests for pharmaceutical-related information. Based on the difficulty and futility that I experienced in obtaining information from Health Canada under the Freedom of Information Act, and in comparison, the relative ease and helpfulness of the FDA, I plan on researching how both countries' systems of public access to information function and why they vary. Undoubtedly, there is much to learn about, and in the very least, raise public awareness of, the relative ease and helpfulness with which Health Canada promises to deliver requests as compared to its actual manifestation, and why this is so.

6.3. RELATING TO THE LARGER NETWORK

International comparative studies have been a major area of research on the "science-based" regulation of technological risks and benefits (Abraham & Davis, 2007, p. 400). Inevitably, this has involved deeper examination of the relationships between researchers and "their social, political, and economic contexts because expert scientists and their scientific work are central to the regulation of biotechnology, environmental chemicals, pharmaceuticals, and many other technologies" (Marks, 1999, as cited in Abraham & Davis, 2007, p. 400; see also Abraham & Millstone, 1989; Daemmrich, 2004; Jasanoff, 2005; Kelman, 1981). Scientific and technological developments in the 1980s and 1990s, in combination with some current social and political trends, have put exceptional pressures on current regulatory organizations and make a review of current practices and approaches to regulation and quality control of pharmaceuticals both timely and necessary. The balance between caution and speed in bringing new products to market, and between public and private sector responsibilities, is having to be looked at afresh and raises a wide range of public policy issues.

In this sociohistorical case study, I have expanded on this important body of work by utilizing international comparisons of regulatory data never before analyzed concurrently. As Mol (2002) attested about her own work, I, too, will about mine; this study does not try to chase away doubt, but seeks instead to raise it. It is my opinion that these cases deserved to be investigated because their identification and contents reveal the nature of what users are not told, while also "opening up" new choices to be made about what users should be able to know. I attempted to investigate why federal regulatory agencies on both sides of the border, although in possession of arguably the same evidence on pharmaceutical safety and adverse reactions for each pharmaceutical in question, made completely different decisions regarding the withdrawal of certain pharmaceuticals off the market. For example, pemoline's unfavorable risk–benefit ratio led to its withdrawal in Canada in 1999, while the FDA instead opted for two separate changes to the pemoline label before completely withdrawing the pharmaceutical in 2005. Although the approval of tolcapone came at relatively similar times in both countries, interestingly, withdrawal decisions once again differed owing to increasing concerns over reports of severe hepatotoxicity: Canada chose to withdraw the pharmaceutical within 1 year, while it is still available in the United States 10 years later.

This study has been concerned with how different elements and different perspectives are joined in the creation of sociotechnological networks. Many sociologists would state that the pharmaceutical networks that I have described can be labeled as "micro" (Mol, 2002). It is true that they are local in the sense that they originate from specific manufacturers who submit data to specific departments of specific organizations in order to be used by specific subsets of patients. The big picture in this case is not sketched out. The social organization of health care, long-term developments in the biomedical sciences, the distribution of power, the flow of capital, and the like—all such macrophenomena appear to escape the microsocial framework of this study at first. Following the networks of pemoline and tolcapone has illustrated, however, that in today's market-oriented, profit-driven health care reviewing industry, sources of funding are major actors. This can result in potentially fatal results for some patients when compounds are not screened properly prior to approval by regulatory agencies, when side effects are overshadowed by manufacturers, and when paid researchers are keen on promoting sales of pharmaceuticals and their publications. It appears that we are distancing ourselves from a completely unbiased, patient-centered state of medicine.

This study, although focused specifically on pemoline and tolcapone, poses new crucial questions about the intersection of science, treatment, and capital. Arguably, pharmaceutical manufacturers have become "deeply enmeshed" in the process that determines which pharmaceuticals we use and when and why and how we use them (Greider, 2003, as cited in Loe, 2004, p. 172). Critics, including Marcia Angell, a former editor of the *New England Journal of Medicine*, have argued that the shift from the academic to the commercial sector has given the industry too much control over clinical pharmaceutical-trial design, data analysis, and publishing (Angell, 2000). On a deeper level of analysis, the cases of pemoline and tolcapone expose how the construction and dissemination of "facts" can be undertaken by corporations, particularly regarding scientific evidence submitted to reviewing bodies and for product monographs. Clearly, current safeguards towards unbiased medical information are lacking. Hence, funding may supply scientific support for a pharmaceutical that can then appease regulators and allow sales. Unfortunately this does not bode well for our society and, increasingly, for other societies worldwide.

There are improvements that must be made in order to improve the quality of our current medical system. While there does exist evidence of corporate infiltration at every level of the creation and dissemination of scientific information, ultimately users of this information hold great capacity. Both prescribers and users of pharmaceuticals decide whether to support such corporations. Although it is naïve to state that complete abstinence from pharmaceuticals, many of which we often rely on, is possible, researching, questioning, and speaking out against certain practices of pharmaceutical companies and physicians is not. Who specifically suffers the most from pharmaceutical harm—harm that might be averted if the present system were changed? What if clinical trial results were reported fully or new pharmaceuticals were not pushed with such force? Or what if regulators were simply left to regulate instead of being "proactive partners" with pharmaceutical manufacturers on what are often only marginally safe and effective medicines? (Crister, 2005, p. 201). The most common victims are the young and the aged and, of course, the parents and children who take care of them. Because clinical trials do not tend to focus on such populations (Kmietowicz, 2000), steering a demographic middle course for both marketing and scientific reasons, little is known about how many pharmaceuticals will affect the young and the old. As an article in the journal *Pediatrics* pointed out, "More than 70 percent of all Physicians' Desk Reference entries have either no existing dosing information for pediatric patients or explicit statements that the safety and efficacy in children have not been determined" (Blumer, 1999, p. 598).

What can we do to make the industry more responsible? The answer, in my opinion, is more independent regulation. First and foremost, we must return Health Canada and the FDA to their primary task as mandated by law—that of regulating and overseeing an industry, not being proactive partners with it. In order to do this, we must end, or at least deeply modify, the agency's client-type relationship with pharmaceutical companies (Crister, 2005). Furthermore, in order to fully restore patient-physician trust, we must extend that transparency even further. As a result, we must salvage the reputation of medicine by placing more distance between physicians, both academics and practitioners, and pharmaceutical power. As Crister (2005, p. 242) wrote, "being independent from pharmaceutical influence matters."

It was my goal to both employ and augment the knowledge of public health officials, epidemiologists, health economists, and physicians. My research examining the previously unexplored phenomenon of discrepancies in pharmaceutical withdrawal policies between Canada and the United States is crucial in helping to shape the future of medical treatment and health policy for all Canadians. After all, health, illness, and treatment are fundamentally social concepts rather than purely biophysical ones.

REFERENCES

Abraham, J. (2002a). Making regulation responsive to commercial interests: Streamlining pharmaceutical industry watchdogs. *British Medical Journal, 325,* 1164–1170.

Abraham, J. (2002b). The pharmaceutical industry as a political player. *The Lancet, 360,* 1498–1502.

Abraham, J., & Davis, C. (2005). A comparative analysis of pharmaceutical safety withdrawals in the UK and the US (1971–1992): Implications for current regulatory thinking and policy. *Social Science & Medicine, 61,* 881–892.

Abraham, J., & Davis, C. (2007). Deficits, expectations and paradigms in British and American pharmaceutical safety assessments: Prying open the black box of regulatory science. *Science, Technology & Human Values, 32,* 399–431.

Abraham, J., & Lawton Smith, H. (Eds.). (2003). *Regulation of the Pharmaceutical Industry.* New York City: Palgrave Macmillan.

Abraham, J., & Millstone, E. (1989). Food additive controls: Some international comparisons. *Food Policy, 14,* 43–57.

Adcock, K. G., MacElroy, D. E., Wolford, E. T., & Farrington, E. A. (1998). Pemoline therapy resulting in liver transplantation. *Annals of Pharmacotherapy, 32,* 422–425.

Akrich, M. (1992). The de-scription of technical objects. In W. E. Bijker & John Law (Eds.), *Shaping technology/building society: Studies in sociotechnical change* (pp. 205–224). Cambridge, MA: MIT Press.

Andriola, M. R. (2000). Efficacy and safety of methylphenidate and pemoline in children with attention deficit hyperactivity disorder. *Current Therapeutic Research, 61*, 208–215.

Angell, M. (2000). Is academic medicine for sale? *New England Journal of Medicine, 342*, 1516–1518.

Anonymous. (1992). WHO stresses interest in ICH. *Scrip*, 1708, 18–20.

Anonymous. (1993). ICH2: Status of tripartite harmonisation initiatives. *Scrip*, 1872, 19.

Assal, F., Spahr, L., Hadengue, A., Rubbici-Brandt, L., & Burkhard, P. R. (1998). Tolcapone and fulminant hepatitis. *The Lancet, 352*, 958.

Avorn, J. (2007). Paying for pharmaceutical approvals—Who's using whom? *The New England Journal of Medicine, 356*, 1697–1700.

Baas, H., Beiske, A. G., Ghika, J., Jackson, M., Oertel, W. M., Poewe, W., & Ransmayr, G. (1997). Catechol-*O*-methyltransferase inhibition with tolcapone reduces the "wearing off" phenomenon and levodopa requirements in fluctuating Parkinsonian patients. *Journal of Neurology, Neurosurgery and Psychiatry, 63*, 421–428.

Bakke, O. M., Manocchia, M., de Abajo, F., Kaitin, K. I., & Lasagna, L. (1995). Drug safety discontinuations in the United Kingdom, the United States, and Spain from 1974 through 1993: A regulatory perspective. *Clinical Pharmacology and Therapeutics, 58*, 108–117.

Basara, L. R. (1996). The impact of a direct-to-consumer prescription medication advertising campaign on new prescription volume. *Pharmaceutical Information Journal, 30*, 715–729.

Beach, J. E., Faich, G. A., Bormel, F. G., & Sasinowski, F. J. (1998). Black box warnings in prescription pharmaceutical labelling: Results of a survey of 206 pharmaceuticals. *Food and Pharmaceutical Law Journal, 53,* 403–411.

Berg, M., & Mol, A. (Eds.). (1998). *Differences in Medicine: Unraveling Practices, Techniques, and Bodies.* Durham, NC: Duke University Press.

Berkovitch, M., Pope, E., Phillips, J., & Koren, G. (1995). Pemoline-associated fulminant liver failure: Testing its evidence for causation. *Clinical Pharmacological Therapy, 57,* 696–698.

Blumenthal, D., Campbell, E., Causino, N., & Seashore, L. K. (1996). Participation of life-science faculty in research relationships with industry. *New England Journal of Medicine, 446,* 1743–1739.

Blumenthal, D., Causino, N., Campbell, E., & Seashore, L. K. (1996). Relationships between academic institutions and industry in the life sciences. *New England Journal of Medicine, 334,* 368–374.

Blumer, J. L. (1999). Off-label uses of pharmaceuticals in children. *Pediatrics, 104,* 598–602.

Bodewitz, H. J., Buurma, H., & de Vries, G. H. (1987). Regulatory science and the social management of trust in medicine. In W. E. Bijker, T. P. Hughes, & T. J. Pinch (Eds.), *The social construction of technological systems: New directions in the sociology and history of technology* (pp. 243–259). Cambridge, MA: MIT Press.

Bonaccorso, S. N., & Sturchio, J. L. (2002). Direct to consumer advertising is medicalising normal human experience: Against. *British Medical Journal, 324,* 910–911.

Borges, N. (2003). Tolcapone-related liver dysfunction—Implications for use in Parkinson's disease therapy. *Pharmaceutical Safety*, *26*, 743–747.

Borges, N. (2005). Tolcapone in Parkinson's disease: Liver toxicity and clinical efficacy. *Expert Opinion on Pharmaceutical Safety*, *4*, 69–73.

Borroni, E., Borgulya, J., & Zurcher, G. (1998). Mose Da Prada and the discovery of tolcapone. *Journal of Neural Transmission*, *52*(Suppl.), 13–16.

Borroni, E., Cesura, A. M., Gatti, S., & Gasser, R. (2001). A preclinical re-evaluation of the safety profile of tolcapone. *Functional Neurology*, *16*, 125–134.

Braithwaite, J. (1986). *Corporate crime in the pharmaceutical industry.* London: Routledge.

Brewer, T., & Colditz, G. (1999). Postmarketing surveillance and adverse drug reactions: Current perspectives and future needs. *Journal of the American Medical Association*, *281*, 824–829.

British Columbia Cancer Agency. (2008). *British Columbia Cancer Agency—Care and research.* Retrieved May 12, 2008, from http://www.bccancer.bc.ca/PPI/CancerTreatment/default.htm

Brown, J. S., Kaitin, K. I., McAuslane, N., Thomas, K. E., & Walker, S. R. (1996). Population exposure required to assess clinical safety: Report to the ICH working group. *Pharmaceutical Information Journal*, *30*, 17–27.

Brown, R. T., Freeman, W. S., Perrin, J. M., Stein, M. T., Amler, R. W., & Feldman, H. M. (2001). Prevalence and assessment of attention-deficit/hyperactivity disorder in primary care settings. *Pediatrics*, *107*, 43–54.

Callon, M. (1986). Some elements of a sociology of translation: Domestication of the scallops and the fishermen of St Brieuc Bay. In J. Law (Ed.), *Power, action and belief* (pp. 196–233). London: Routledge & Kegan Paul.

Callon, M., & Latour, B. (1981). Unscrewing the Big Leviathan. In K. D. Knorr-Cetina & A. V. Cicourel (Eds.), *Advances in social theory and methodology: Towards an integration of micro- and macro-sociologies* (pp. 277–303). Boston: Routledge & Kegan Paul.

Carpenter, D., Zucker, E. J., & Avorn, J. (2008). Drug-review deadlines and safety problems. *The New England Journal of Medicine, 358*, 1354–1361.

Castillo, J., Fabrega, E., Escalante, C. F., Sanjuan, J. C., Herrera, L., & Hernanz, F. (2001). Liver transplantation in a case of steatohepatitis and subacute hepatic failure after biliopancreatic diversion for morbid obesity. *Obesity Surgery, 11*, 640–642.

Center for Drug Evaluation and Research. (1998). *The CDER Handbook*. Rockville, MD: The Food and Drug Administration. Retrieved December 4, 2008, from http://www.fda.gov/cder/handbook/

Center for Drug Evaluation and Research, Medical Reviews. (1998). *Regarding new drug application (Tasmar)* (pp. 10, 46). Rockville, MD.

Center for Responsive Politics Web site. (2008, June 8). *Pharmaceutical manufacturing*. Retrieved June 11, 2008, from http://www.opensecrets.org/lobby/induscode.php?lname=H4300&year=2008

Cho, M. K., & Bero, L. A. (1996). The quality of pharmaceutical studies published in symposium proceedings. *Annals of Internal Medicine, 235*, 485–489.

Colosimo, C. (1999). The rise and fall of tolcapone. *Journal of Neurology, 246*, 880–882.

Conrad, P., & Leiter, V. (2004). Medicalization, markets and consumers. *Journal of Health and Social Behavior, 45*, 158–176.

Crister, G. (2005). *Generation Rx: How prescription pharmaceuticals are altering American lives, minds and bodies.* Boston: Houghton Mifflin Company.

Cylert Product Monograph. (1984). *Pemoline (Cylert).* Abbott Park, Illinois: Abbott Laboratories, Inc.

Daemmrich, A. (2004). *Pharmacopolitics: Pharmaceutical regulation in the United States and Germany.* Chapel Hill: University of North Carolina Press.

Da Prada, M., Keller, H. H., Pieri, L., Kettler, R., & Haefely, W. E. (1984). The pharmacology of Parkinson's disease: Basic aspects and recent advances. *Experientia, 40*, 1165–1172.

D'Arcy, P. F., & Harron, D. W. G. (Eds.). (1998). *Proceedings of the fourth international conference on harmonisation.* Belfast, U.K.: IFPMA.

Davidson, R. A. (1986). Source of funding and outcome of clinical trials. *Journal of General Internal Medicine, 2*, 155–158.

de Laet, M., & Mol, M. (2000). The Zimbabwe bush pump. *Social Studies of Science. 30*, 225–263.

Department of Health and Human Services. (n.d.). *Tasmar tablets—Misleading claims* [letter] (NDA #20-697). Rockville, MD: Author.

Department of Health and Human Services. (1998a). *Division of Pharmaceutical Marketing, Advertising and Communications— Violative promotional materials for Tasmar (tolcapone) tablets* (NDA 20-697). Rockville, MD: Author.

Department of Health and Human Services. (1998b). *List of drug products that have been withdrawn or removed from the market for reasons of safety or effectiveness* (21 CFR Part 216, [Docket No. 98N-0655]). Rockville, MD: Food and Drug Administration.

Department of Health and Human Services. (2001). *Division of Pharmaceutical Marketing, Advertising and Communications— Violative promotional materials for Tasmar (tolcapone) tablets* (NDA 20-697). Rockville, MD: Food and Drug Administration.

Division of Neuropharmacological Drug Products—Food and Drug Administration (U.S.). (1997). *Supervisory review of NDA 20-697, Tasmar, an adjunct to l-dopa treatment in patients with Parkinson's disease* (NDA 20-697, p. 1). Rockville, MD: Centre for Drug Evaluation and Research.

Elitsur, Y. (1990). Pemoline (Cylert)-induced hepatotoxicity. *Journal of Pediatric Gastroenterological Nutrition, 11*, 143–144.

Entacapone to Tolcapone Switch Study Investigators, The. (2007). Entacapone to tolcapone switch: Multicenter double-blind, randomized, active-controlled trial in advanced Parkinson's disease. *Movement Disorders, 22*, 14–19.

Epstein, S. (1996). *Impure science: AIDS, activism, and the politics of knowledge*. Los Angeles: University of California Press.

European Medicines Agency. (2004). *Committee for medicinal products for human use: European public assessment report (EPAR) for Tasmar* (EMEA/H/C/132). London: European Medicines Agency.

Factor, S. A., Molho, E. S., Feustel, P. J., Brown, D. L., & Evans, S. M. (2001). Long-term comparative experience with tolcapone and entacapone in advanced Parkinson's disease. *Clinical Neuropharmacology, 24,* 295–299.

Fleck, L. (1981). *Genesis and development of a scientific fact.* Chicago, IL: University of Chicago Press.

Food and Drug Administration. (1974, March 15). *Pharmacologist review of NDA 16-832, NDA original amendment of February 2, 1974.* Rockville, MD: Author.

Food and Drug Administration. (1999a). *CDER New Molecular Entity Approvals in Calendar Year 1999.* Retrieved November 30, 2008, from http://www.fda.gov/cder/rdmt/nmecy99.htm

Food and Drug Administration. (1999b, January 11). *The Food and Drug Administration: An overview.* Retrieved November 29, 2008, from http://www.cfsan.fda.gov/fdaoview.html

Food and Drug Administration. (2005a). *Immediately remove from the market pemoline, Cylert-Abbott Laboratories, and all generic versions, a stimulant pharmaceutical for the treatment of attention deficit hyperactivity disorder.* Retrieved October 2006, from http://www.fda.gov/ohrms/dockets/dockets/05p 0115/05p0115.htm

Food and Drug Administration. (2005b). Liver injury risk and market withdrawal. *Alert for healthcare professionals.* Retrieved December 4, 2008, from http://www.fda.gov/Cder/drug/InfoSheets/HCP/pemolineHCP.htm

Food and Drug Administration—Centre for Drug Evaluation and Research. (2008). *Drugs @ FDA—Drug details—Tasmar.* Retrieved March 20, 2008, from http://www.accessdata.fda.gov/scripts/cder/drugsatfda/index.cfm?fuseaction=Search. DrugDetails

40. 63 *Federal Register* 195. (1998). (codified at 21 CFR).

Freeman, R. D. (1976). *Minimal brain dysfunction, hyperactivity, and learning disorders: Epidemic or episode?* Chicago: University of Chicago Press.

Friedman, M. A., Woodcock, J., Lumpkin, M. M., Shuren, J. E., Hass, A. E., & Thompson, L. J. (1999). The safety of newly approved medicines: Do recent market removals mean there is a problem? *Journal of the American Medical Association, 281,* 1728–1734.

Fuller, S. (2000). Why science studies has never been critical of science: Some recent lessons on how to be a helpful nuisance and a harmless radical. *Philosophy of the Social Sciences, 30,* 5–32.

Gale, E. A. (2001). Lessons from the glitazones: A story of pharmaceutical development. *Lancet, 357,* 1870–1875.

Garutti, R. J. (1994). Clinical safety data management: Definitions and standards for expedited reporting. In P. F. D'Arcy & D. W. G. Harron (Eds.), *Proceedings of the second international conference on harmonisation* (pp. 376–382). Belfast, U.K.: IFPMA.

Gomart, E. (2002). Methadone: Six effects in search of a substance. *Social Studies of Science, 32,* 93–135.

Goozner, M. (2004). *The $800 million pill: The truth behind the cost of new pharmaceuticals.* Los Angeles: University of California Press.

Gordon, A. J. (1994). Clinical safety data management: Definitions and standards for expedited reporting. In P. F. D'Arcy & D. W. G. Harron (Eds.), *Proceedings of the second international conference on harmonisation* (pp. 384). Belfast, U.K.: IFPMA.

Graham, D., Campen, D., Hui, R., Spence, M., Cheetham, C., & Levy, G. (2005). Risk of acute myocardial infarction and sudden cardiac death in patients treated with cyclo-oxygenase 2 selective and non-selective non-steroidal anti-inflammatory drugs: Nested case-control study. *The Lancet, 365*, 475–481.

Greenhill, L. L. (2000, May 18). *Evidence-based stimulant treatments for ADHD.* Paper presented at the 123rd meeting of the American Psychiatric Association, Chicago.

Greider, K. (2003). *The big fix: How the pharmaceutical industry rips off American Consumers.* New York: Public Affairs Publishers.

Guthrie, P. (2007). US senate passes FDA revitalization act. *Canadian Medical Association Journal, 177*, 23.

Haasio, K., Sopanen, L., Vaalavirta, L., Linden, I. B., & Heionen, E. H. (2001). Comparative toxicological study on the hepatic safety of entacapone and tolcapone in the rat. *Journal of Neural Transmission, 108*, 79–91.

Harris, G. (2007, June 27). Psychiatrists top list in pharmaceutical maker gifts. *New York Times*, p. A14.

Harris, G., & Berenson, A. (2005, February 25). 10 voters on panel backing pain pills had industry ties. *New York Times*, p. A1.

Health Canada. (1999). *Therapeutic Products Programme's international strategy* (International Policy Division). Ottawa, Ontario: Health Canada.

Health Canada. (2000). Pemoline (Cylert): Market withdrawal. *Canadian Adverse Drug Reaction Newsletter, 10*, 2.

Health Canada. (2006a). *Access to therapeutic products—The regulatory process in Canada* (Health Products and Food Branch). Ottawa, Ontario: Health Canada.

Health Canada. (2006b). *Product life cycle*. Retrieved November 30, 2008, from http://www.hc-sc.gc.ca/sr-sr/biotech/health-prod-sante/prod_life-vie-eng.php

Health Canada. (2007). *The progressive licensing framework concept*: *Paper for discussion*. Retrieved December 3, 2008, from http://www.hc-sc.gc.ca/dhp-mps/homologation-licensing/develop/proglic_homprog_concept-eng.php

Health Canada. (2008). *Patent register—Entacapone*. Retrieved November 30, 2008, from http://205.193.93.51/patent/english/record_results.cfm?din_number=02243763&patent_number=2342634&term=Entacapone

Health Canada Advisory. (1998, November 23). *Liver complications reported with anti-Parkinson's pharmaceutical TASMAR*. Ottawa, Ontario: Health Canada. Retrieved June 21, 2007, from http://www.hc-sc.gc.ca/ahc-asc/media/advisories-avis/1998-eng.php

Health Canada Advisory. (1999). *Liver complication results in withdrawal of attention deficit hyperactivity disorder pharmaceutical, Cylert* (1999-113). Ottawa, Ontario: Health Canada.

Hébert, P. C. (2007). Progressive licensing needs progressive open debate. *Canadian Medical Association Journal, 176*, 1801.

Hennessy, S., & Strom, B. L. (2007). PDUFA reauthorization—Pharmaceutical safety's golden moment of opportunity? *New England Journal of Medicine, 356*, 1703–1704.

Hess, D. J. (1997). *Science studies: An advanced introduction*. New York: New York University Press.

Hochman, J. A., Woodard, S. A., & Cohen, M. B. (1998). Exacerbation of autoimmune hepatitis: Another hepatotoxic effect of pemoline therapy. *Pediatrics, 101*, 106–108.

Hoffmann-La Roche Laboratories. (1998). *Important pharmaceutical warning*. Nutley, NJ: Hoffmann-La Roche Laboratories, Inc.

Hogan, V. (2000). Pemoline (Cylert): Market withdrawal. *CMAJ: Canadian Medical Association Journal, 162,* 106.

Holmstrom, J., & Stalder, P. M. (2001). Drifting technologies and multi-purpose networks: The case of the Swedish cashcard. *Information and Organization, 11,* 187–206.

Honein, M. A., Paulozzi, L. J., & Erickson, J. D. (2001). Continued occurrence of Accutane-exposed pregnancies. *Teratology, 64,* 142–147.

Human Resources Development Canada. (2002). *Prevalence of hyperactivity-impulsivity and inattention among Canadian children: Findings from the first data collection cycle (1994–1995) of the National Longitudinal Survey of Children and Youth* (SP-561-01-03E). Hull, Quebec: Human Resources Development Canada Publications Centre.

Hurwitz, M. A., & Caves, R. E. (1988). Persuasion or information? Promotion and the shares of brand name and generic pharmaceuticals. *The Journal of Law and Economics, 31,* 299–320.

Idanpaan-Heikkila, J. (1998). Impact and implementation of the ICH guidelines. In P. F. D'Arcy & D. W. G. Harron (Eds.), *Proceedings of the fourth international conference on harmonisation* (pp. 33–34). Belfast, U.K.: IFPMA.

Immen, W. (1998, December 11). Hyperactivity drug under study, on sale. *The Globe and Mail,* p. A13.

International Conference on Harmonisation. (1995). *Guideline on the need for carcinogenicity studies of pharmaceuticals.* Geneva, Switzerland: IFPMA.

Jaffe, S. L. (1989). Pemoline and liver function. *Journal of the American Academy of Child and Adolescent Psychiatry, 28,* 457–458.

Jasanoff, S. (2005). *Designs on nature: Science and democracy in Europe and the United States.* Princeton, NJ: Princeton University Press.

Jones, M. I., Greenfield, S. M., & Bradley, C. P. (2001). Prescribing new pharmaceuticals: Qualitative study of influences on consultants and general practitioners. *British Medical Journal, 323,* 378–381.

Kaledin, M. (Medical Correspondent). (2005, February 25). Was painkiller panel stacked? 10 members of committee that ok'd Cox-2 pills had drug company ties [Television series episode]. In *Medical News.* New York City: CBS.

Kaplan, B., Truex, D. P., Wastell, D., Wood-Harper, A. T., & DeGross, J. I. (Eds.). (2004). *Information systems research—Relevant theory and informed practice.* Norwell, MA: Kluwer Academic Publishers.

Keating, G. M., & Lyseng-Williamson, K. A. (2005). Tolcapone—A review of its use in the management of Parkinson's disease. *CNS (Central Nervous System) Pharmaceuticals, 19,* 165–184.

Kelly, L., Lazzaro, M., & Petersen, C. (2007). Canadian pharmaceutical regulatory framework. *The Canadian Journal of Neurological Sciences, 34*(Suppl. 1), S3–S10.

Kelman, S. (1981). *Regulating America, regulating Sweden: A comparative study of occupational safety and health policy.* Cambridge, MA: MIT Press.

Keung, N., & Daly, R. (1998, December 9). Parents renew call for inquest doctor prescribed pharmaceutical to boy, 14, without warning about side effects. *The Toronto Star,* p. A23.

Kieburtz, K., & Hubble, J. (2000). Benefits of COMT inhibitors in levodopa-treated Parkinsonian patients: Results of clinical trials. *Neurology*, *55*(Suppl. 4), S42–S45.

Klecun, E. (2004). Conducting critical research in IS: Can actor-network theory help? In B. Kaplan, D. P. Truex, D. Wastell, A. T. Wood-Harper, & J. I. DeGross (Eds.), *Information systems research—Relevant theory and informed practice* (pp. 259–274). Norwell, MA: Kluwer Academic Publishers.

Kmietowicz, Z. (2000). Pharmaceutical industry is unwilling to run trials in children. *The British Medical Journal*, *320*, 1362.

Knowles, F. (2005, October 25). Abbott's ADD pharmaceutical loses FDA backing. *The Chicago Sun-Times*, p. 62.

Kondro, W. (2002). Pharmaceutical approvals taking too long? *Canadian Medical Association Journal*, *166*, 790.

Kondro, W. (2007). Health Canada proposes new regulatory regime for pharmaceuticals. *Canadian Medical Association Journal*, *176*, 1261–1262.

Konopka, M., & Czlonkowski, A. (2005). Comparison of the safety of the medicinal product in the European Union and the United States, tolcapone (Tasmar)—COMT inhibitor as the analyzed example. *Neurologia i Neurochirurgia*, *39*, 490–496.

KPMG Consulting LP. (2000, June 16). *Report volume 1: Review of the Therapeutic Products Programme cost recovery initiative*. Ottawa, Ontario: Ministry of Health.

Kurth, M. C., Adler, C. H., St. Hilaire, M., Singer, C., Waters, C., LeWitt, P., et al. (1997). Tolcapone improves motor function and reduces levodopa requirement in patients with Parkinson's disease experiencing motor fluctuations: A multicenter, double-blind, randomized, placebo-controlled trial. *Neurology, 48,* 81–87.

Laine, C., Horton, R., DeAngelis, C. D., Godlee, F., Drazen, J. M., & Frizelle, F. A. (2007). Clinical trial registration: Looking back and moving ahead. *The Lancet. 177,* 57–58.

Lasser, K. E., Allen, P. D., Woolhandler, S. J., Himmelstein, D. U., Wolfe, S. M., & Bor, D. H. (2002). Timing of new black box warnings and withdrawals for prescription medications. *Journal of the American Medical Association, 287,* 2215–2220.

Latour, B. (1987). *Science in Action.* Cambridge, MA: Harvard University Press.

Latour, B. (1993). *We have never been modern.* Cambridge, MA: Harvard University Press.

Latour, B. (1994). On technical mediation—Philosophy, sociology, genealogy. *Common Knowledge, 3,* 29–64.

Latour, B. (1996). The trouble with actor-network theory. *Philosophia, 25,* 47–64.

Latour, B. (1999). *Pandora's hope.* Cambridge, MA: Harvard University Press.

Latour, B. (2004). On using ANT for studying information systems: A (somewhat) Socratic dialogue. In C. Averou, C. Ciborra, & F. Land (Eds.), *The social study of information and communication technology: Innovation, actors and contexts* (pp. 252–279). Oxford: Oxford University Press.

Latour, B. (2005). *Reassembling the social.* London: Oxford University Press.

Latour, B., & Woolgar, S. (1979). Laboratory life: The construction of scientific facts. Princeton, NJ: Princeton University Press.

Law, Jacky. (2006). Big pharma: How the world's biggest pharmaceutical companies control illness. London: Constable & Robinson Ltd.

Law, John. (1991). A sociology of monsters: Essays on power, technology and domination. London: Routledge.

Law, John. (1999). After ANT: Complexity, naming and topology. In J. Law & J. Hassard (Eds.), Actor network theory and after (pp. 1–14). Oxford: Blackwell Publishers/The Sociological Review.

Law, John. (2001). Networks, relations and cyborgs: On the social study of technology. Lancaster University Centre for Science Studies and the Department of Sociology. Retrieved November 28, 2008 from http://www.lancs.ac.uk/fass/sociology/papers/law-networks-relations-cyborgs.pdf

Law, John, & Callon, M. (1992). The life and death of an aircraft: A network analysis of technical change. In W. E. Bijker & J. Law (Eds.), Shaping technology/building society: Studies in sociotechnical change (pp. 21–52). Cambridge, MA: MIT Press.

Law, John, & Mol, A. (1995). Notes on materiality and sociality. The Sociological Review, 43, 274–294.

Lazarou, J., Pomeranz, B., & Corey, P. N. (1998). Incidence of adverse drug reactions in hospitalized patients: A meta-analysis of prospective studies. The Journal of the American Medical Association, 279, 1200–1205.

Lee, N., & Brown, S. D. (1994). Otherness and the actor network. *American Behavioral Scientist*, 37, 772–791.

Leegwater-Kim, J., & Waters, C. (2006). Tolcapone in the management of Parkinson's disease. *Expert Opinion on Pharmacotherapy*, 7, 2263–2270.

Lexchin, J. (1984). *The real pushers—A critical analysis of the Canadian pharmaceutical industry*. Vancouver: New Star Books.

Lexchin, J. (2004). New directions in pharmaceutical approval. *Canadian Medical Association Journal*, 171, 229– 230.

Lexchin, J. (2005). Pharmaceutical withdrawals from the Canadian market for safety reasons, 1963–2004. *Canadian Medical Association Journal*, 172, 765–767.

Lexchin J. (2006a). A comparison of new pharmaceutical availability in Canada and the United States and potential therapeutic implications of differences. *Health Policy*, 79, 214–220.

Lexchin, J. (2006b). Relationship between pharmaceutical company user fees and pharmaceutical approvals in Canada and Australia: A hypothesis-generating study. *The Annals of Pharmacotherapy*, 40, 2216–2222.

Lienert, G. A., & Janke, W. (1957). Pharmakopsychologische untersuchung uber 5-phenyl-2-imino-4-oxo-oxazolidin. *Arzneimittel-Forschung*, 7, 436–439.

Lipsky, M. S., & Sharp, L. K. (2001). From idea to market: The pharmaceutical approval process. *Journal of the American Board of Family Practitioners*, 14, 362–367.

Loe, M. (2004). *The rise of Viagra: How the little blue pill changed sex in America.* New York: New York University Press.

Lucas, C. J., & Knowles, J. B. (1963). The trial of a new stimulant, pemoline, in the treatment of fatigue in students. *Journal of the American College Health Association, 12,* 187–194.

Lurie, P. (2006). Financial conflicts of interest are related to voting patterns at FDA advisory committee meetings. *Medscape General Medicine, 8,* 22.

Lurie, P., Almeida, C. M., Stine, N., Stine, A. R., & Wolfe, S. M. (2006). Financial conflict of interest disclosure and voting patterns at Food and Drug Administration pharmaceutical advisory committee meetings. *Journal of the American Medical Association, 295,* 1921–1928.

Lyles, A. (2002). Direct marketing of pharmaceuticals to consumers. *Annual Review of Public Health, 23,* 73–91.

Macinnes, A. (1997). Central Europe working towards ICH standards. *Scrip.* 2279, 60.

Maguire, P. (1999, March). How direct-to-consumer advertising is putting the squeeze on physicians. *ACP-ASIM Observer.* Retrieved March 9, 2008 from http://www.acpinternist.org/archives/1999/03/squeeze.htm

Marks, L. (1999). "Not just a statistic": The history of USA and UK policy over thrombotic disease and the oral contraceptive pill, 1960s–1970s. *Social Science & Medicine, 49,* 1139–1155.

Marotta, P. J., & Roberts, E. A. (1998). Pemoline hepatotoxicity in children. *Journal of Pediatrics, 132,* 894–897.

Marra, C. A., Lynd, L. D., Anis, A. H., & Esdaile, J. M. (2006). Approval process and access to prescription pharmaceuticals in Canada. *Arthritis & Rheumatism (Arthritis Care & Research)*, *55*, 9–11.

Mather, C. M. (2005). The pipeline and the porcupine: Alternate metaphors of the physician-industry relationship. *Social Science & Medicine*, *60*, 1323–1334.

Mather, C. M. (2006). Medical innovation, unmet medical need, and the pharmaceutical pipeline. *Canadian Journal of Clinical Pharmacology*, *13*, 85–91.

McCurry, L., & Cronquist, S. (1997). Pemoline and hepatotoxicity. *American Journal of Psychiatry*, *154*, 713–714.

McKinlay, J. B. (1981). From "promising report" to "standard procedure": Seven stages in the career of a medical innovation. *Milbank Memorial Fund Quarterly/Health and Society*, *59*, 374–411.

Meadley, R. G. (1965). A new anti-fatigue agent in general practice. *The Practitioner*, *195*, 680–683.

Meadows, M. (2001, May). Serious liver injury: Leading reason for pharmaceutical removals, restrictions. *FDA Consumer Magazine*, *35*, 5–8.

Medicines Control Agency. (1997). Volital (pemoline) has been withdrawn. *Current Problems in Pharmacovigilance*, *23*, 9–12.

Miller, H. (2007, March 14). National experts and nonprofit organizations urge major changes to "FDA reform" legislation. Retrieved February 29, 2008, from http://www.center4research.org/news/fda-press-release-03-07.html

Mintzes, B., Barer, M. L., Kravitz, R. L., Bassett, K., Lexchin, J., Kazanjian, A., Evans, R. G., Pan, R., & Marion, S. A. (2002). Influence of direct to consumer pharmaceutical advertising and patients' requests on prescribing decisions: Two site cross sectional survey. *British Medical Journal, 324*(7332), 278–279.

Mol, A. (2002). *The body multiple: Ontology in medical practice.* Durham, NC: Duke University Press.

Montaner, J., O'Shaughnessy, M., & Schechter, M. (2001). Industry-sponsored clinical research: A double-edged sword. *Lancet.* 358, 1893–1895.

Monteiro, E. (2000). Actor-network theory and information infrastructure. In C. Ciborra (Ed.), *Control to drift* (pp. 71–83). New York: Oxford University Press.

Morgan, S. G. (2007). Direct-to-consumer advertising and expenditures. *Open Medicine, 1,* e37–e45.

Mosholder, A. (2006). The Food and Drug Administration— Pediatric Advisory Committee. *Psychiatric adverse events in attention deficit hyperactivity disorder (ADHD) in clinical trials.* PowerPoint presentation given for the Pediatric Advisory Committee Meeting. FDA Division of Drug Risk Evaluation.

Moynihan, R., & Cassels, A. (2005). *Selling sickness—How the world's biggest pharmaceutical companies are turning us all into patients.* Vancouver: Douglas & McIntyre Publishing Group.

Murdoch, J. (2001). Ecologising sociology: Actor-network theory, co-construction and the problem with human exemptionalism. *Sociology,* 35, 111–133.

Murphy, M. N., Smith, M. C., & Juergens, J. P. (1992). The synergic impact of promotion intensity and therapeutic novelty on market performance of prescription pharmaceutical products. *Journal of Pharmaceutical Issues, 22,* 305–316.

Myers, A., & Moore, S. R. (1987). The drug approval process and the information it provides. *Pharmaceutical Intelligence & Clinical Pharmacy, 21,* 821–826.

Nakajima, H. (1996). The ICH programme: Accomplishments and impact on world health. In P. F. D'Arcy & D. W. G. Harron (Eds.), *Proceedings of the Third International Conference on Harmonisation* (p. 32). Belfast, U.K.: IFPMA.

Nehra, A., Mullick, F., Ishak, K. G., & Zimmerman, H. J. (1990). Pemoline-associated hepatic injury. *Gastroenterology, 99,* 1517–1519.

Nissen, S. E., & Wolski, K. (2007). Effect of rosiglitazone on the risk of myocardial infarction and death from cardiovascular causes. *New England Journal of Medicine, 356,* 2457–2471.

Obeso, J. A., Rodriguez-Oroz, M. C., Chana, P., Lera, G., Rodriguez, M., & Olanow, C. W. (2000). The evolution and origin of motor complications in Parkinson's disease. *Neurology, 55,* S13–S20.

Page, J. G., Bernstein, J. E., Janicki, R. S. & Michelli, F. A. (1974). A multi-clinic trial of pemoline in childhood hyperkinesis. In C. K. Conners (Ed.), *Clinical use of stimulant pharmaceuticals in children.* Proceedings of a symposium held at Key Biscayne, Florida, March 5–8, 1972 (pp. 98–124). New York: Exerpta Medica.

Patterson, J. F. (1984). Hepatitis associated with pemoline. *Southern Medical Journal, 77,* 938.

Peay, M. Y., & Peay, E. R. (1988). The role of commercial sources in the adoption of a new pharmaceutical. *Social Science of Medicine, 26,* 1183–1189.

Petersen, M. (2000, October 5). Pushing pills with piles of money: Merck and Pharmacia in arthritis pharmaceutical battle. *New York Times*, C:1.

Pharmaceutical Research and Manufacturers of America. (2002). *PHRMA annual report 2001–2002*. Washington, DC: Pharmaceutical Research and Manufacturers of America.

Pickering, A. (1992). *Science as practice and culture*. Chicago: University of Chicago Press.

Pirmohamed, M., Breckenridge, A. M., Kitteringham, N. R., & Park, B. K. (1998). Adverse drug reactions. *British Medical Journal*, 316, 1295–1298.

Pizzuti, D. (1996). *Black box warning letter, Cylert*. Abbott Park, IL: Abbot Laboratories.

Pizzuti, D. (1999). *Revised black box warning, Cylert*. Abbott Park, IL: Abbot Laboratories.

Pliszka, S. R. (1998). The use of psychostimulants in the pediatric patient. *Child and Adolescent Psychopharmacology, 45*, 1085–1098.

Polanczyk, G., de Lima, M. S., Horta, B. L., Biederman, J., & Rohde, L. A. (2007). The worldwide prevalence of ADHD: A systematic review and metaregression analysis. *American Journal of Psychiatry, 164*, 942–948.

Pratt, D. S., & Dubois, R. S. (1990). Hepatotoxicity due to pemoline (Cylert): A report of two cases. *Journal of Pediatric Gastroenterology and Nutrition, 10*, 239–241.

Prout, A. (1996). Actor-network theory, technology and medical sociology: An illustrative analysis of the metered dose inhaler. *Sociology of Health and Illness, 18*, 198–219.

Psaty, B. M., Furberg, C. D., Ray, W. A., & Weiss, N. S. (2004). Potential for conflict of interest in the evaluation of suspected adverse pharmaceutical reactions—Use of cerivastatin and risk of rhabdomyolysis. *The Journal of the American Medical Association, 292*, 2622–2631.

Public Citizen's Health Research Group. (2001). *Study of the pharmaceutical industry's performance in finishing required postmarketing research (Phase IV) studies* (HRG Publication #1520). Washington, DC: Public Citizen Press Office.

Public Citizen's Health Research Group. (2005). *Letter to FDA urging the immediate recall of all outstanding supplies of generic pemoline from the market* (HRG Publication #1754). Washington, DC: Public Citizen Press Office.

Rajput, A. H., Martin, W., Saint-Hilaire, M. H., Dorflinger, E., & Peder, S. (1997). Tolcapone improves motor function in Parkinsonian patients with the "wearing off" phenomenon: A double-blind, placebo-controlled, multicenter trial. *Neurology, 49*, 1066–1071.

Rawson, N., & Kaitin, K. (2003). Canadian and US drug approval times and safety considerations. *The Annals of Pharmacotherapy, 37*, 1403–1408.

Rawson, N. S. (2005). Assessing prescription medications for priority regulatory review. *Regulatory Toxicology and Pharmacology, 42*, 70–76.

Rosenberg, S. A. (1996). Secrecy in medical research. *New England Journal of Medicine, 445*, 392–394.

Rosh, J. R., Dellert, S. F., Narkewich, M., Birnbarum, A., & Whittington, G. (1998). Four cases of severe hepatotoxicity associated with pemoline: Possible autoimmune pathogenesis. *Pediatrics, 101,* 921–923.

Ross, D. B. (2007). The FDA and the case of Ketek. *The New England Journal of Medicine, 356,* 1601–1604.

Safer, D. J., & Zito, J. M. (2000). The pharmacoepidemiology of Ritalin. In L. L. Greenhill & B. B. Osman (Eds.), *Ritalin: Theory and patient management* (2nd ed., pp. 7–26). Larchmont, NY: Liebert.

Safer, D. J., Zito, J. M., & Gardner, J. F. (2001). Pemoline hepatotoxicity and postmarketing surveillance. *Journal of the American Academy of Child and Adolescent Psychiatry, 40,* 622–629.

Singleton, V., & Michael, M. (1993). Actor-networks and ambivalence: General practitioners in the U.K. cervical cancer screening programme. *Social Studies of Science.* 23, 227–264.

Skerritt, J. (2007, June 12). Avandia concerns spark call for reforms: Pharmaceutical-approval process endangers patients, experts say. *Winnipeg Free Press,* p. A2.

Stalder, F. (2000). Beyond constructivism: Towards a realist realism: A review of Bruno Latour's Pandora's hope. *The Information Society, 16,* 245–247.

Star, S. L. (1991). Power, technologies and the phenomenology of conventions: On being allergic to onions. In J. Law (Ed.), *A sociology of monsters? Essays on power, technology and domination, vol. 38. Sociological review monograph* (pp. 26–56). London: Routledge.

Steinbrook, R. (2005). Financial conflicts of interest and the Food and Drug Administration's advisory committees. *New England Journal of Medicine, 353,* 116–118.

Stelfox, H. T., Chua, G., O'Rourke, K., & Detsky, A. S. (1998). Conflict of interest in the debate over calcium-channel antagonists. *New England Journal of Medicine, 449*, 101–106.

Sterling, M. J., Kane, M., & Grace, N. D. (1996). Pemoline-induced autoimmune hepatitis. *American Journal of Gastroenterology, 91*, 2233–2234.

Stipp, D., & Moore, A. H. (1998). Impotence is a much bigger problem than doctors used to think, and new pills are on the way to treat it. *Fortune, 137*(5) 114–123.

Stross, J. K. (1987). Information sources and clinical decisions. *Journal of General Internal Medicine, 2*, 155–159.

Talland, G. A., & McGuire, M. T. (1967). Tests of learning and memory with Cylert. *Psychopharmacologia, 10*, 445–451.

Tasmar Product Monograph. (1998). Tolcapone (Tasmar). Nutley, NJ: Hoffmann-La Roche Laboratories, Inc.

Tasmar Product Monograph. (2006). Tolcapone (Tasmar). Nutley, NJ: Hoffmann-La Roche Laboratories, Inc.

Thompson, L. (2000). User fees for faster drug reviews—Are they helping or hurting the public health? *FDA Consumer Magazine.* Retrieved December 2, 2008, from http://www.fda.gov/Fdac/features/2000/500_pdufa.html

Waknine, Y. (2006, May 24). FDA safety changes: Ability, Fortamet, Tasmar. *Medscape Medical News.* Retrieved June 21, 2007, from http://www.medscape.com/viewarticle/533065

Walker, S. R., & Lumley, C. E. (1987). Reporting and underreporting. In R. D. Mann (Ed.), *Adverse drug reactions: The scale and nature of the problem and the way forward* (pp. 115–126). Carnforth, U.K.: Parthenon.

Walsham, G. (1997). Actor-network theory and IS research: Current status and future prospects. In A. S. Lee, J. Liebenau, & J. I. DeGross (Eds.), *Information systems and qualitative research* (pp. 466–480). London: Chapman & Hall.

Watkins, P. (2000). COMT inhibitors and liver toxicity. *Neurology, 55*(Suppl. 4), S51–S52.

Wilens, T. E., Biederman, J., Spencer, T., Frazier, J., Prince, J., & Bostic, J. (1999). Controlled trial of high doses of pemoline for adults with attention-deficit/hyperactivity disorder. *Journal of Clinical Psychopharmacology, 19*, 257–264.

Williams-Jones, B., & Graham, J. E. (2003). Actor-network theory: A tool to support ethical analysis of commercial genetic testing. *New Genetics and Society, 22*, 271–296.

Willman D. (2000, December 20). How a pharmaceutical policy led to seven deadly pharmaceuticals. *Los Angeles Times*, A:1.

Willy, M. E., Manda, B. M., Shatin, D., Drinkard, C. R., & Graham, D. J. (2002). A study of compliance with FDA recommendations for pemoline (Cylert). *Journal of the American Academy of Child and Adolescent Psychiatry, 41*, 785–790.

Wood, S. (2007, March 14). *Scholars issue open letter on FDA reform*. Retrieved February 29, 2008, from http://www. defendingscience.org/newsroom/PDUFA-open-letter.cfm

Yeates, N., Lee, D. K., & Maher, M. (2007). Health Canada's progressive licensing framework. *Canadian Medical Association Journal, 176*, 1845–1847.

Young, A. (1981). When rational men fall sick: An inquiry into some assumptions made by medical anthropologists. *Culture, Medicine and Psychiatry, 5*, 317–335.

INDEX

www.ingramcontent.com/pod-product-compliance
Lightning Source LLC
Chambersburg PA
CBHW070426270326
41926CB00014B/2966